THE
PLASTIC
SURGERY
SOURCEBOOK

THE PLASTIC SURGERY SOURCEBOOK

EVERYTHING YOU NEED TO KNOW

KIMBERLY A. HENRY, M.D.

AND

PENNY HECKAMAN

AFTERWORD BY
CAROLYN J. CLINE, M.D., PH.D.

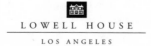

LOWELL HOUSE

LOS ANGELES

CONTEMPORY BOOKS

CHICAGO

Library of Congress Cataloging-in-Publication Data

Henry, Kimberly A., 1959-
    The plastic surgery sourcebook : everything you need to know / Kimberly A. Henry and
Penny Heckaman.
        p.   cm.
    Includes bibliographical references and index.
    ISBN 1-56565-464-1
    1.Surgery, Plastic—Popular works.   2. Consumer education.
    I. Heckaman, Penny.   II. Title.
RD119.H46   1996
    617.9'5—dc21
                                                     96-49696
                                                          CIP

Requests for such permissions should be addressed to:
Lowell House
2020 Avenue of the Stars, Suite 300
Los Angeles, CA 90067

Lowell House books can be purchased at special discounts when ordered in bulk for premiums and special sales. Contact Department TC at the address above.

Publisher: Jack Artenstein
Associate Publisher, Lowell House Adult: Bud Sperry
Managing Editor: Maria Magallanes
Text design: Laurie Young

Illustrations by Sandy Nern/Studio 8 Graphics and Khosrow Matini, M.D.
Photographs courtesy of Kimberly A. Henry, M.D., Edward Terino, M.D., Carolyn J. Cline,
M.D., Ph.D., Khosrow Matini, M.D., Miguel Delgado, M.D., Dudley Cheu, D.D.S., Sam Ray,
Barry Schwartz, M.D., Lifecell Corporation, Collagen Corporation, and Coherent Laser
Corporation

Manufactured in the United States of America
10 9 8 7 6 5 4 3 2 1

To our kids—
Jenny and Andrew
Alexandra, Adam, Brooke, and Lisa

ACKNOWLEDGMENTS

We would like to thank several professionals, organizations, and friends for their support and contributions to this book.

The editors, Maria Magallanes and Bud Sperry, and the publisher, Jack Artenstein

The American Society of Plastic and Reconstructive Surgeons, especially Nancy Ryan from the Communications Department

The Aesthetic Society

The United States Department of Agriculture

The United States Department of Health and Human Services

Linda Decker, transcriptionist extraordinare

Derek Gallagher

Duane Newcomb, literary consultant for Newcomb & Newcomb Literary Agency

Dudley Cheu, D.D.S.

Carolyn J. Cline, M.D.

Miguel Delgado, M.D.

Khosrow Matini, M.D.

Sandy Nern, Studio 8 Graphics

Sam Ray, tattoo artist

Ed Terino, M.D.

Pamela Jeffrey

Debbie Lindsey

Maggie Tucker

Sarah Brown

Mindy Brown

Mickey and Bill Henry

Mark Gorney, M.D.

Barry Schwartz, M.D.

Lifecell Corporation

Coherent Laser Corporation

Collagen Corporation

CONTENTS

So You're Thinking About Plastic Surgery

Remember all those mornings when you relied on the good old alarm clock and that first sip of strong coffee to wake you up? As the years went by, did you find that after you turned off the alarm, a good look in the mirror was stronger than any Colombian coffee? Unfortunately, there's nothing like the cold, cruel, reality of the morning light on a naked, sleepy face to wake up practically anyone!

If you have been having these "meaningful mirror encounters" as of late, it has probably occurred to you that things aren't quite where they used to be but are actually much further south! Have "gravity grooves" set in? Well, join the group. The baby boomers have hit forty and fifty and are quickly making their way to plastic surgery offices everywhere.

It happens to everyone, we are all vain, and we would all like to look and feel better. So, if it's possible to change the things we can, why not? Wouldn't it be terrific to look into the mirror and see a face that isn't sagging, wrinkling, and tired-looking; a neck that is firmer and one that actually goes back and in from the chin to the neck; and eyes that look refreshed and rested—but still have character. Imagine breasts that are full and toned; an abdomen that doesn't exactly look like a nineteen-year-old's, but then doesn't look like your last two pregnancies were for baby elephants either; thighs that are firm and in proportion; and calves and ankles that are smooth, fat-free, and do not resemble tree stumps.

Are we dreaming here? Is all of this possible? Can you really feel so good about yourself again? The answer is yes, you can. The purpose of this book is to help you understand as much as possible about plastic surgery from your initial visit with the doctor all the way to the "new, younger and fresher-looking you." We will describe what you should experience during various appointments with your surgeon and explain different surgical procedures. And, we'll tell you the truth. You'll learn what to expect before, during, and after your procedure, as well as information on average costs, statistics, hospitals, surgery centers, special post-surgery garments, possible risks and complications, nonsurgical procedures, and more. We will show you how to pick a board certified plastic surgeon in your area who is trained to do the particular procedure you are interested in.

This is the first book about plastic surgery that presents a point of view that you can understand. We hope to provide you with a clear perspective on what you will go through from beginning to end. Hopefully, this book will be a source of information and comfort, as well as pleasant hours of reading. Our main goal is to prepare you for plastic surgery each step of the way. But, we also hope that by reading a book written in a relaxed, down-to-earth manner (like chatting about a face-lift over a latte with your best friend), you will feel comfortable about the whole process of plastic surgery and what it has to offer you. We feel that the more informed the prospective patient is, the more positive his or her experience will be. Since I have undergone plastic surgery procedures myself, I understand what a patient will go through, how they will feel, and their fears and concerns.

This book has been designed and written to inform you and also to entertain. After all, you have the opportunity to change physical characteristics that could make you feel better about your appearance, that could make you feel better about yourself. You can explore all your possibilities in a relaxed, casual atmosphere that will be more interesting and fun than reading another dry, dull medical book.

So, enjoy the book and, hopefully, it will prepare you for your surgery. We will begin with the initial consultation with the surgeon and give you a step-by-step guide throughout the entire process. But first, you will need to ask yourself if plastic surgery is right for you.

CHAPTER 1

IS PLASTIC SURGERY FOR YOU?

Elective plastic surgery is becoming increasingly popular every year, and thousands of procedures are performed all over the world and on all types of people. Magazines are filled with articles on the subject, and society's pressures to look young, thin, healthy, and beautiful influence would-be patients to think seriously about plastic surgery. Have you seen the face or body of your dreams jump out at you from some glossy journal and decide then and there that surely a plastic surgeon could make you look like that? *Reality check!*

Photos can certainly help when you're discussing your goals and expectations with a surgeon, but you must also be realistic. The people whose faces and bodies you're craving from magazines and advertisements were actually born with 80 percent of what you see. The height, bone structure, and weight tendency (although there has been much speculation about the so-called diets of models) are pretty much a genetic gift to these lucky few. So, it would be unreasonable to go to a surgeon and say, "I want to look exactly like a supermodel," when your one thigh is practically the size of both of her hips! However, a photo can give the doctor some idea of the look you would like, and after examining you, the surgeon will determine whether your goals are achievable.

One of the most important things you can ask yourself is, "Am I considering cosmetic surgery for me or to please someone else in my life?" It is crucial for a candidate of plastic surgery to understand that surgery should never be considered to please your husband or wife, boyfriend or girlfriend, employers or co-workers. It should be done for you and you alone. A change in your face, eyes, nose, or body can boost your self-confidence, self-esteem, and will greatly affect how you project yourself to the world. Often, a patient who has had a breast augmentation finds herself standing up straighter, walking more self-assuredly, and marveling at how great she looks and feels in her clothes. Your significant other, friends, and family will, of course, be the grateful beneficiaries of a happy, refreshed "new" you. But, what you've done for yourself and your outlook on life will, hopefully, be the best present you can give yourself. So, it is important to analyze your reasons for contemplating a change in your appearance.

On a piece of paper write down the name of the procedure you're thinking about having. Then, underneath the type of surgery write one column that says PROS and another that says CONS. Be totally honest with yourself and list your arguments both for and against having the procedure. Normal reasons under the CONS column might be: cost, time away from work, anticipated child care, and fear of physical change or discomfort. However, if you've listed things like: your family wouldn't approve, your friends say your nose is just fine, or your boyfriend will leave you if you change your looks, then these are definitely not reasons for you to cancel your plans for surgery.

Under the PROS column, normal reasons would be: you would feel and look younger, your clothes would fit better, your self-esteem should improve, and you would probably project yourself to the world in a more self-confident, comfortable manner. But, if you've listed things like: my boyfriend will be more attracted to me if my breasts are larger, or I'll certainly get a promotion at work if I change my nose and look prettier, or my dating life will skyrocket after I have liposuction, then you should not be considering plastic surgery. These are the thoughts of an insecure person with low self-esteem, who feels that by changing her looks the world will suddenly become perfect.

Remember, changing your outer appearance will not change who you are inside. It will not solve problems with boyfriends or automatically put you in contention for the vice-presidency of your company. It may, however, result in greater self-confidence and a sense of security about yourself, thereby enriching many aspects of your life. Sometimes, it is helpful to consult with a psychologist or counselor if you are unclear about your decision to have plastic surgery.

Before we discuss various procedures such as face-lifts or nose surgery, we'd like to explain a little about the field of plastic surgery so that you have a better understanding of what it involves as well as its history.

CHAPTER 2

PLASTIC SURGERY—
A DEFINITION AND HISTORY

We restore, repair, and make whole those parts
which nature has given but fortune has taken away,
not so much to delight the eye, but to buoy up the spirit
and help the mind of the afflicted.

—GASPAR TAGLIACOZZI,
FATHER OF PLASTIC SURGERY
1596 A.D.

This quote from almost five hundred years ago is a perfect definition of plastic surgery—a medical specialty that has distinct branches of its own. The word *plastic* is derived from the ancient Greek word *plastikos,* which means to mold or give form. Plastic surgery includes both the reconstructive and aesthetic subspecialties, and it is the latter branch upon which we will be concentrating.

Plastic, or reconstructive, surgery deals with correcting deformities and disfigurements caused by birth defects, injury, or disease. Examples of such operations are the rebuilding of amputated or deformed arms or legs; repairing cleft lips, badly-formed noses and ears; and reconstructing a breast after mastectomy. A badly-burned patient will usually seek the services of a plastic surgeon to repair the damaged skin, as will those patients with scars or birthmarks. These patients can benefit from techniques such as skin-grafting, in which tissue is taken from one part of the body and is then used on another. Tissue transplantation is actually the "essence" of plastic surgery.

One of the oldest of the surgical specialties, many of the methods used today can be traced back to medical writings dating several centuries B.C. The American Society of Plastic and Reconstructive Surgeons (ASPRS) states, "Because human beings have always sought self-fulfillment through self-improvement, plastic surgery—improving and restoring form and function—may be one of the world's oldest healing arts." In fact, written evidence suggests that physicians in ancient India used skin grafts in reconstructive surgery as early as 3300 B.C. During this time, plastic surgery was a necessity for persons caught committing adultery and whose tops of their noses were cut off as a consequence. Noses were then fashioned out of forehead skin. This procedure, developed 3300 years ago, is still being done today. But progress in this field moved slowly, and it wasn't until the nineteenth and twentieth centuries that major developments were made in this area in Europe and the United States.

America's first plastic surgeon was Dr. John Peter Mettauer, born in Virginia in 1787, and a leader in the first cleft palate operation in 1827. But the main event that brought about most plastic surgery developments was World War I. Suddenly, doctors needed to treat extensive facial and head wounds, destroyed noses, and gaping wounds caused by the war.

In another quote from the ASPRS, aesthetic, or cosmetic, surgical procedures also developed during this period as physicians realized, in the words of nineteenth-century American plastic surgeon John Orlando Roe, "How much valuable talent had been buried from human eyes, lost to the world and society by reason of embarrassment caused by the conscious, or in some cases, unconscious influence of some physical infirmity or deformity or unsightly blemish."

By World War II, many plastic surgeons served in the armed service treating wounded soldiers, sailors, and airmen. New foundations were formed, and scientific journals were written especially for surgeons in this specialty. The most important one, in 1946, was the *Journal of Plastic and Reconstructive Surgery*—the official publication of the ASPRS. This journal has been a source of knowledge and new discoveries for doctors throughout the years.

By the 1950s, plastic surgery fully moved into the medical establishment and the public eye by way of radio and television appearances. New discoveries were happening very quickly, some of which were used during the Korean War.

In the 1960s, Americans became interested in any information about the

Table 2-1.
1992 National Plastic Surgery Statistics
(Top Five Procedures Indicated in Bold)

Procedure	Total	Plastic Surgery Procedures % of Total
Birth defects	33,501	2.2
Breast augmentation (Augmentation mammoplasty)	32,607	2.1
Breast lift (Mastopexy)	7,963	.5
Breast reconstruction	29,607	1.9
Breast reduction	39,639	2.6
Breast reduction in men (Gynecomastia)	4,997	.3
Burn care	17,552	1.1
Buttock lift	291	*
Cheek implants (Malar augmentation)	1,741	.1
Chemical peel	19,049	1.2
Chin augmentation (Mentoplasty)	4,115	.2
Collagen injections	41,623	2.7
Dermabrasion	13,457	.9
Dog bites	10,376	.7
Ear surgery (Otoplasty)	6,371	.4
Eyelid surgery (Blepharoplasty)	**59,461**	**3.9**
Face-lift (Rhytidectomy)	40,077	2.6
Fat injections	7,865	.5
Forehead lift	13,501	.9
Hand surgery	**138,233**	**9.1**
Lacerations	**135,494**	**8.9**
Liposuction (Suction-assisted lipectomy)	47,212	3.1
Male-pattern baldness	1,955	.1
Maxillofacial surgery	22,095	1.5
Microsurgery	19,405	1.3
Nose reshaping (Rhinoplasty)	50,175	3.3
Retin-A treatment	23,520	1.5
Scar revision	**52,647**	**3.5**
Subcutaneous mastectomy	2,458	.2
Thigh lift	1,023	*
Tummy tuck (Abdominoplasty)	16,810	1.1
Tumor removal	**502,567**	**33.2**
Other aesthetic	1,098	*
Other reconstructive	116,737	7.7
Total	1,515,222	100

* Denotes less than 0.1 percent.
+ All figures are projected, based on a survey of ASPRS members only.

Reprinted with permission of the American Society of Plastic and Reconstructive Surgeons.

newest cosmetic procedures. In 1962, silicone, a new substance used to treat skin imperfections, was first used in a breast implant device. The American public was ready to try such an exciting new experiment. Further notice was given to this specialty during the Vietnam War when ASPRS member Dr. Hal Jennings was appointed United States Surgeon General, the first and only plastic surgeon to achieve this public service honor.

By the 1970s, the forty-five-year-old ASPRS had grown from a handful of New York doctors to nearly two thousand members across the country, and plastic surgery had come into its own in the medical profession. In the 1980s, the leaders of the specialty wanted to bring more knowledge to the public, so the ASPRS began producing a large amount of brochures on various surgical procedures.

By the 1990s, more than five thousand board certified plastic surgeons were active in the United States. However, the American public still fails to realize that these surgeons perform reconstructive work as well, and the myth that a plastic surgeon is only a "cosmetic surgeon" perpetuates. In fact, the current ASPRS president, Elvin Zook, M.D., has made changing this perception one of his main goals by suggesting that the name of the society be shortened to the "American Society of Plastic Surgeons." He hopes people will understand that plastic and reconstructive surgeons are the same.

During the 1990s, this medical specialty caught the eye of the public when breast implant safety was questioned. According to scientific information gathered from ASPRS, "Despite the efforts of the (Plastic Surgery) Society to address growing fears in 1991, the Food and Drug Administration severely restricted the use of silicone gel implants in January of 1992." Since then, many studies about the safety of silicone have been conducted, and the use of saline implants are now recommended.

Research continues in this highly specialized branch of surgery to develop new ideas and improve new techniques for patients. The ASPRS has offered a list of statistics on plastic surgery for use in this book. Please refer to Table 2-1.

Aesthetic, or cosmetic, surgery, is the focus of this book. These types of procedures are elective, ones we choose to do. It is not life-threatening to have small breasts, a crooked nose, or sagging jowls, so, a patient might choose to undergo elective surgery to correct such a problem.

This type of plastic surgery includes procedures intended to correct, add, or reduce certain features that make the patient unhappy or that are medically required. For example, a droopy eyelid can make you look tired, sad, and older—not the look of choice for most people. A blepharoplasty, or eye surgery, is the procedure done to correct this. However, at the same time, the eyelid droops so much that it can obstruct eyesight, and make surgery medically necessary. We will discuss this further in Chapter 10.

It's amazing how some people are perfectly happy with unusual characteristics while others are racing off to the surgeon's office. A good example of this is Cindy Crawford's mole. While most people want to have moles removed and feel that they are blemishes on their otherwise acceptable faces and bodies, Cindy appears to be marketing her mole quite well—even emphasizing it with certain positions and camera angles. Everyone feels differently about things such as moles, but some people, like Miss Crawford, are perfectly content (and often proud) of their "unusual" trademarks. It's the other million people who make appointments with plastic surgeons to permanently get rid of what's bothering them. Many other procedures are performed by the plastic surgeon to help these patients, but we only list a few. In later chapters, we will discuss various procedures in depth, so that you will understand more about your chosen surgery.

In this book, we will refer to the physician as a plastic surgeon, since most doctors in this specialty have been trained in all branches of plastic, reconstructive, and aesthetic (or cosmetic) surgery. We will explain many common surgical procedures, most of which you are probably familiar with, and some of which you are not.

Please refer to this list of terms when you speak to your doctor, or simply for your own personal information:

Rhinoplasty: Nose surgery
Rhytidectomy: Face-lift
Blepharoplasty: Eyelid surgery
Brow lift: Lifts brows and forehead
Mastopexy: Breast lift
Abdominoplasty: Tummy tuck
Liposuction: Suction-assisted fat removal
Augmentation mammoplasty: Saline or silicone implant to enlarge a breast
Genioplasty: Chin contouring
Reduction mammoplasty: Reducing a large breast
Malar augmentation: Cheek implant
Breast reconstruction: Creating a new breast
Laser resurfacing: Using laser to improve wrinkles

The plastic surgeon also performs several non-surgical procedures such as chemical peels, dermabrasion, and hair transplants.

It is most important that you, the prospective surgical patient, understand and be prepared for the fact that the surgeon must prepare you for all aspects of your procedure. The doctor will counsel you and prepare you emotionally before any surgery can be performed, stressing the importance of realistic expectations and goals, and informing you of any risks or complications.

If you're considering plastic surgery, you might be interested in reading some statistics for procedures performed during the last few years. This information was provided by the American Society of Plastic and Reconstructive Surgeons and includes figures for nearly all categories of plastic surgery procedures. Although we will basically concentrate on cosmetic or aesthetic procedures in this book, it is interesting to see a list of all types of surgery in this field. You will find some surprising figures in the appendices located at the end of this book. For instance, plastic surgeons perform reconstructive procedures nearly three times as often as aesthetic procedures. It is also interesting to find that eye surgery (blepharoplasty) was performed more often than any other cosmetic or aesthetic plastic surgery.

Among procedures generally classified as reconstructive, the most often performed was tumor removal. This was actually performed more often than any other plastic surgery procedure, with more than 400,000 performed in 1994.

Reconstructive procedures outnumber those classified as aesthetic nearly three to one. Total reconstructive procedures total nearly 1 million, while procedures typically considered aesthetic total nearly 393,000. In 1993, members of the ASPRS removed breast implants in more than 25,000 patients, including implants that were originally placed for reconstructive as well as cosmetic reasons.

James Wells, M.D., former ASPRS Public Education Chair, said, "Recent ASPRS surveys have shown that the average plastic surgeon's practice is made up of more than 60 percent reconstructive procedures."

At the same time, nearly 40,000 women opted to have breast augmentation in 1992, more than 90 percent of these with saline-filled implants. Approximately another 22,800 women received implants for reconstruction after disease or mastectomy.

About 13 percent of all aesthetic surgery patients are men, while teenagers (those eighteen years old and younger) make up about 4 percent of aesthetic

Table 2-2.
1994 Reconstructive Procedures
(Top Five Procedures Indicated in Bold)

Procedure	Total	Reconstructive Procedures % of Total
Birth defects	15,318	1.6
Breast implant removal	9,198	.9
Breast reconstruction	25,933	2.6
Breast reduction	**36,074**	**3.7**
Burn care	13,814	1.4
Dog bites	10,050	1.0
Hand surgery	**144,308**	**14.7**
Lacerations	**114,303**	**11.7**
Maxillofacial surgery	14,152	1.4
Microsurgery	15,942	1.6
Scar revision	**35,809**	**3.7**
Subcutaneous mastectomy	1,423	.1
Tumor removal	**431,417**	**44.0**
Other reconstructive	112,269	11.5
Total	**980,010**	**100.0**

Reprinted with permission of the American Society of Plastic and Reconstructive Surgeons.

surgery patients. The most popular procedure with men was nose reshaping, with eye surgery and liposuction next. Teens most often requested nose reshaping.

Statistics show that people undergoing plastic surgery represent a wide spectrum of society—executives, baby boomers, senior citizens, professionals, and teens. Magazines and newspapers regularly feature articles on the subject, and studies have shown that plastic surgery is no longer a luxury reserved for the very rich. According to the ASPRS, some 30 percent of people choosing plastic surgery have family incomes of less than $25,000 a year. About 35 percent have incomes between $25,000 and $50,000, and only 23 percent earn more than $50,000.

The statistics suggest that you are certainly not alone in your quest for improvement. Even though the lists show figures from a few years back, they are the most current and up-to-date that the ASPRS could provide. Compiling the numbers takes a great deal of time by the members who record all of the procedures performed throughout the year. These facts are then sent to the ASPRS Public Education Chair for accurate compilation.

We'd like to thank the ASPRS for their generous contribution to this chapter. The American Society of Plastic and Reconstructive Surgeons represents 97 percent of all physicians certified by the American Board of Plastic Surgery, the only board recognized by the American Board of Medical Specialties to certify in plastic surgery. Consumers may call the Plastic Surgery Information Service at 1-800-635-0635 for brochures and a list of qualified plastic surgeons in their area.

Table 2-3.
1994 Aesthetic and Reconstructive Procedures
(Top Five Procedures Indicated in Bold)

Procedure	Total	Aesthetic Procedures % of Total
Breast augmentation	**39,247**	**10.0**
Breast implant removal	28,655	7.3
Breast lift	10,053	2.6
Breast reduction in men	4,416	1.1
Buttock lift	314	*
Cheek implants	1,136	.3
Chemical peel	29,072	7.4
Chin augmentation	3,632	.9
Collagen injections	27,052	6.9
Dermabrasion	10,100	2.6
Ear surgery	4,684	1.2
Eyelid surgery	**50,838**	**12.9**
Face-lift	**32,283**	**8.2**
Fat injections	9,038	2.3
Liposuction	**51,072**	**13.0**
Male-pattern baldness	2,571	.7
Nose reshaping	**35,927**	**9.1**
Retin-A treatment	20,875	5.3
Thigh lift	1,098	.3
Tummy tuck	16,829	4.3
Upper arm lift	633	.2
Wrinkle injection	342	*
Total	**393,049**	**100**

*Denotes less than 0.1 percent

Reprinted with permission of the American Society of Plastic and Reconstructive Surgeons.

CHAPTER 3

How Much Is This Going to Cost Me?

How Do I Pick a Plastic Surgeon?

If you don't already know it, plastic surgery is not cheap. In fact, it's quite expensive, and because it is usually your decision to have cosmetic, or elective, surgery, insurance companies will not cover these procedures. Also, plastic surgeons commonly require that you pay them for their services in full beforehand. In some cases, however, a financial payment plan can be arranged either in the form of a loan through the American Society of Plastic and Reconstructive Surgeons or through a personal financing plan agreed to by your individual doctor.

Costs for plastic surgery, the physician's fees, and hospital and surgery center charges vary from one region of the country to another. A lot has to do with the cost of living factor and the surgeon's personal fee scale. Fees near or in major metropolitan areas such as Chicago, New York, or San Francisco can be much higher than those for the same procedures done in Duluth or Des Moines.

There are certain instances when an insurance carrier will cover some expenses of plastic surgery. In cases of trauma when surgery is necessary due to an accident, or if a congenital malformation such as a cleft lip is present, the procedure will most likely be taken care of by the insurance company. For the most part, because cosmetic surgery is not life-threatening or medically necessary, the patient

Table 3-1.
1992 Average Surgeon Fees*

Procedure	National Average	CA	NY	FL	TX
Breast augmentation	$2,754	$3,141	$3,522	$2,756	$2,718
Breast lift	3,063	3,385	4,010	3,113	2,970
Breast reconstruction					
Implant alone	2,340	2,719	2,885	2,468	2,444
Tissue expander	2,846	2,881	3,561	3,204	2,999
Latissimus dorsi	4,509	4,536	5,395	5,147	5,031
TRAM (pedicle) flap	6,143	5,187	7,483	6,489	6,209
Microsurgical free flap	6,758	5,685	6,692	7,262	6,711
Breast reduction	4,525	4,929	5,432	5,293	4,515
Breast reduction in men	2,325	2,687	3,061	2,470	2,026
Buttock lift	3,084	2,798	5,120	3,175	3,566
Cheek implants	1,895	1,870	2,654	1,701	1,530
Chemical peel					
Full face	$1,634	$1,849	$2,217	$1,668	$1,454
Regional	682	762	869	711	626
Chin augmentation					
Implant	1,221	1,380	1,907	1,153	901
Osteotomy	2,077	2,342	2,990	2,133	1,413
Collagen injections-per 1cc	266	296	328	278	259
Dermabrasion	1,551	1,840	2,267	1,486	1,344
Ear surgery	2,098	2,216	2,822	2,198	2,074
Eyelid surgery					
Both uppers	1,514	1,601	1,939	1,469	1,524
Both lowers	1,519	1,633	2,151	1,447	1,478
Combination of both	2,625	2,784	3,594	2,564	2,593
Face-lift	4,156	4,448	5,410	4,026	4,148
Fat injection					
Head/Neck	636	702	695	717	695
Trunk	622	571	794	645	300
Extremities	663	572	794	644	689
Forehead lift	2,164	2,484	3,207	2,002	1,852
Liposuction-any single site	1,622	2,028	2,346	1,603	1,563
Male-pattern baldness					
Plug grafts-per plug	101	162	152	297	23
Strip grafts-per strip	1,096	869	1,500	1,150	1,200

*Fees generally range according to region of country and patient needs. These fees are averages only.

Continued on next page

Table 3-1—*Continued*

Procedure	National Average	CA	NY	FL	TX
Scalp reduction-all stages	1,720	2,549	2,357	2,084	1,350
Pedicle flap-all stages	2,699	5,308	2,525	3,067	1,600
Tissue expansion-all stages	3,081	3,609	4,175	3,244	2,000
Nose reshaping (primary)					
Fee for open rhinoplasty	2,997	3,390	4,371	2,947	3,019
Fee for closed rhinoplasty	2,825	3,131	4,160	2,705	2,689
Nose reshaping (secondary)					
Fee for open rhinoplasty	2,615	3,130	3,426	2,806	2,662
Fee for closed rhinoplasty	2,649	2,958	3,841	2,819	2,525
Retin-A treatment-per visit	92	56	83	58	39
Thigh lift	3,090	3,093	4,723	3,115	3,098
Tummy tuck	3,618	4,085	4,774	3,754	3,581

Reprinted with permission of the American Society of Plastic and Reconstructive Surgeons.

takes full responsibility for any expenses. In some cases, however, the surgery may be covered by insurance. Examples include a rhinoplasty as a result of the correction of a deviated septum, a blepharoplasty if a sagging eyelid restricts vision, breast reconstruction after mastectomy, and breast reduction when the patient has suffered from neck, shoulder, and back pain due to extremely large breasts.

Refer to Table 3-1 for cosmetic surgery charges, and understand that these are average fees and may vary depending upon where you have your surgery done. Once again, the figures reflect the national and regional averages. Tables 3-2 and 3-3 reflect sample costs for a hospital and surgery center. (Be aware that these facilities are all in the San Francisco Bay Area and reflect the higher cost of living in Northern California.)

Of course, before embarking on plans for any surgical procedure, be sure to get the total cost information for your doctor's services, the hospital or surgery center's fees, and any extra costs that may be added. After all, what good is a beautiful new face or body if you've gone into a state of shock when the final bill arrives?

After much soul-searching about whether or not to have plastic surgery, a crash course in its definition and history, and the shocking realization that your new look could have a price tag equal to two month's salary—you're ready for the next step: selecting a surgeon, a decision that's right up there with your choices regarding a job, home, car, and anything else that will have a major impact on your life.

Table 3-2.
Hospital Charges for Plastic Surgery Procedures

Suggested surgeries for Classes (may change based on patient needs and length of O.R. time). "Class" refers to the time frame involved for the surgery and varies at different locations; "local/standby" means that a local anesthetic is used, usually administered by the doctor with an anesthesiologist standing by if more anesthesia is needed; "general" means that a general anesthetic is used, and the patient is asleep for the entire procedure. These fees are in addition to the surgeon's fees.

Class Number & Surgery Type	Anesthesia Type	Price
Class I: Up to 1 hour	Local	$576
	With Anesthesia	$792
a. Scar revision		
b. Minor suction lipoplasties		
c. Upper and lower blepharoplasty		
d. Coronal lift		
e. Cheek or chin implant		
f. Tip rhinoplasty		
Class II: 1 to 2½ hours	Local	$864
	With Anesthesia	$1,080
a. Augmentation and mammoplasty		
b. Mastopexy		
c. Upper and lower blepharoplasty		
d. Limited face-lift		
e. Rhinoplasty or septo-rhinoplasty		
f. Major suction lipoplasty		
g. Otoplasty		
h. Abdominoplasty		

Continued on next page

Table 3-2—*Continued*

Class Number & Surgery Type	Anesthesia Type	Price
Class III: 2½ to 4 hours	Local	$1,296
	With Anesthesia	$1,776
a. Breast reduction (non-insurance covered)		
b. Face-lift		
c. Face-lift with upper or lower blepharoplasty		
d. Face-lift with coronal lift		
Class IV: over 4 hours	Local	$1,728
	With Anesthesia	$2,160
a. Face-lift, upper & lower lids & coronal lift		
b. Multiple procedure combinations		
One overnight stay:		$300

(first night only; additional nights charged at hospital rates)

- Rates are for cash pay no less than 48 hours in advance & non-insurance covered only.
- Does *not* include:

Lab	EKG	Postoperative or take-home medications
X ray	Implants	Suction lipectomy garments
		Appliances, e.g., braces, splints, etc.

These fees are based on average figures only.

Table 3-3.
Plastic Surgery Procedure Base Times/Charges at a Surgery Center

Procedure	Average time		Fees
Abdominoplasty	3	hours	$ 850
Abdominoplasty with abdominal liposuction	4	hours	950
Abdominoplasty with body liposuction	5	hours	1,100
Blepharoplasty, U or L	1 ½	hours	550
Blepharoplasty, U or L, with brow lift	3	hours	850
Blepharoplasty, U & L	2	hours	625
Blepharoplasty, U & L, with brow lift	4	hours	900
Brachioplasty	2	hours	650
Breast augmentation			
Unilateral	1 ½	hours	500
Bilateral	2	hours	650
Breast implant repositioning (capsulotomy)			
Unilateral	1 ½	hours	475
Bilateral	2	hours	650
Breast mastectomy			
Unilateral	2	hours	650
Bilateral	4	hours	900
Breast mastopexy	2	hours	750
Breast reduction	3	hours	1,000
Brow lift	2 ½	hours	700
Chin implant	1 ½	hours	600
Dermabrasion			600
Fat grafting	1	hour	525
Genioplasty			1,000
Gynecomastia excision with liposuction	2	hours	650
Hematoma evacuation			
Facial	1 ½	hours	550
Breast	1 ½	hours	475
Lip resection	1	hour	600
Malar implant	1 ½	hours	550
Otoplasty	2	hours	650
Rhinoplasty	2 ½	hours	700
Rhinoplasty with septoplasty	3	hours	800
Rhytidectomy (face-lift)	4	hours	900
Rhytidectomy-mini	2	hours	725

Continued on next page

Table 3-3—*Continued*

Procedure	Average time		Fees
Rhytidectomy with brow lift	5	hours	$1,100
Rhytidectomy with facial liposuction	4	hours	950
Rhytidectomy with U or L blepharoplasty	4	hours	950
Rhytidectomy with U & L bleph & brow lift	6	hours	1200
Rhytidectomy with U & L blepharoplasty	5	hours	1,100
Scalp reduction	1	hour	550
Scar revision	2	hours	650
Scar revision with flap graft	3	hours	800
Septoplasty	2 ½	hours	700
Suction minor (one area)	1 ½	hours	600
Suction major (more than one area)	2 ½	hours	750
Thigh lift	3	hours	800
Tip rhinoplasty	2	hours	650
Anesthesia			
(per hour for the first 4 hours)			250
(per hour beginning with the fifth hour)			200

These fees are based on average figures only.

How Do I Pick a Plastic Surgeon

How do you find the right plastic surgeon? How do you know that you will have the same goals and expectations? Is there any guarantee that the surgeon you select will be the answer to your prayers? The only way to get the answers to these questions is to actually meet with the potential candidate in a professional consultation.

You must be careful when choosing your doctor. One reason is that there are no laws to control the training and qualifications of doctors. In fact, anyone who has a medical degree can call themselves a specialist and obtain a license that allows him or her to practice any type of medicine, including plastic surgery. So, doctors who advertise as plastic surgeons may not have actually studied the specialty sufficiently.

According to *A Delineation of Qualifications for Clinical Privilege,* a publication distributed by the American Society of Plastic and Reconstructive Surgeons (October 1994): "In the United States, physicians are generally licensed as *medical practitioners* by state licensing boards. Federal laws do not govern the quality of specialty training or dictate the procedures a physician may aspire to perform. In effect, a medical school graduate can legally claim to be a specialist of his or her choosing with or without residency training in that specialty."

If your doctor is permitted to perform surgery at your hospital you can safely assume that the hospital considers the doctor properly trained in procedures. However, some doctors who have their own surgical suites can legally perform whatever procedure they wish, without other doctors or hospital administrators monitoring them. These are the doctors that you need to watch out for, and it is important for you to check out the doctor's qualifications, training, and experience.

An important thing to look for in your search for a plastic surgeon is that he or she is certified by the American Board of Plastic Surgery (a member of the American Board of Medical Specialties) or an equivalent board, such as the American Board of Facial Plastic Sugery, or that he or she is board qualified (in practice for at least two full years, has taken and passed the board's written exams, and is preparing for, or has taken, the oral exams). Surgeons who meet the requirement of this board are then granted board certification—designating them as diplomates of the American Board of Plastic Surgery. The previously quoted work by the ASPRS also states: "The intent of the certification process, as defined by the member boards of the American Board of Medical Specialties is: to provide assurance that a certified medical specialist has successfully completed an approved educational program and an evaluation including an examination process designed to assess the knowledge, experience, and skills requisite to the provision of high quality patient care in that specialty."

An ENT cosmetic surgeon is a physician who has had training in ear, nose, and throat surgery and, in addition, one or two years in facial plastic surgery training. This surgeon is trained only for face-lift, eye, and nose surgery. Plastic surgeons have four years of general surgery training and two to three years of plastic surgery training. A plastic surgeon can perform a majority of the procedures.

Table 3-4 explains the educational requirements necessary for a doctor to specialize in plastic surgery.

Table 3-4.
Training of the Plastic Surgeon

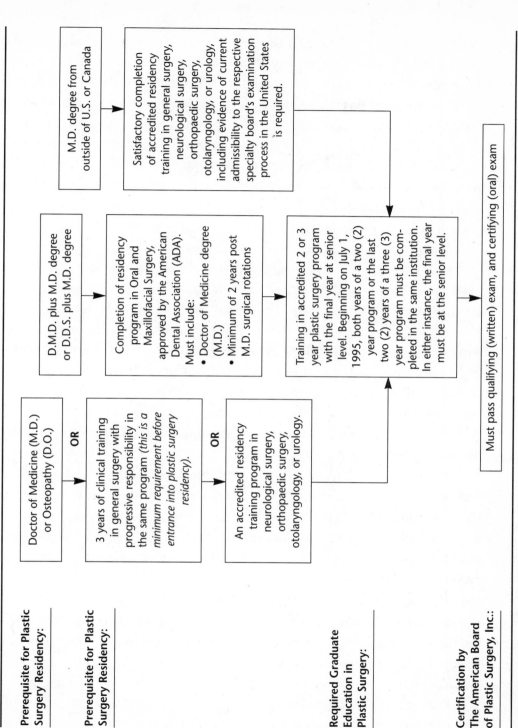

Prerequisite for Plastic Surgery Residency:

Doctor of Medicine (M.D.) or Osteopathy (D.O.)

D.M.D. plus M.D. degree or D.D.S. plus M.D. degree

M.D. degree from outside of U.S. or Canada

Prerequisite for Plastic Surgery Residency:

OR

3 years of clinical training in general surgery with progressive responsibility in the same program (*this is a minimum requirement before entrance into plastic surgery residency*).

OR

An accredited residency training program in neurological surgery, orthopaedic surgery, otolaryngology, or urology.

Completion of residency program in Oral and Maxillofacial Surgery, approved by the American Dental Association (ADA).
Must include:
• Doctor of Medicine degree (M.D.)
• Minimum of 2 years post M.D. surgical rotations

Satisfactory completion of accredited residency training in general surgery, neurological surgery, orthopaedic surgery, otolaryngology, or urology, including evidence of current admissibility to the respective specialty board's examination process in the United States is required.

Required Graduate Education in Plastic Surgery:

Training in accredited 2 or 3 year plastic surgery program with the final year at senior level. Beginning on July 1, 1995, both years of a two (2) year program or the last two (2) years of a three (3) year program must be completed in the same institution. In either instance, the final year must be at the senior level.

Certification by The American Board of Plastic Surgery, Inc.:

Must pass qualifying (written) exam, and certifying (oral) exam

Reprinted with permission of the American Society of Plastic and Reconstructive Surgeons.

As you can see, even before the doctor is in a position to take the board exams to become a diplomate, he or she will have completed many years of specialty training in plastic surgery. To become certified at the end of training, the doctor must pass a written, or qualifying, exam and an oral, or certifying, exam. Certification means that the physician has completed the training and practice necessary to perform plastic surgery. Some doctors further their education through added experience such as a fellowship, a three- to twelve-month training program either in a hospital or with an individual doctor. Plastic surgeons may also earn a CAQ (Certificate of Added Qualification) in hand surgery. It is important to remember that once a doctor is certified in plastic surgery, he has been highly trained in the specialty and has been evaluated by his peers on his practice.

Now that you know how much work and training the plastic surgeon needs to complete to get where he is, find one who is a good match for you. The first step in your search for "Dr. Right" is to call the American Society of Plastic and Reconstructive Surgeons for a list of recommended doctors in your area. You can request a doctor who specializes in one procedure, such as a face-lift, a doctor who is geographically desirable, a male or female, or one who has operating privileges at your preferred hospital or surgery center. You may ask as many questions as you like, since this process may help you narrow down your choices of a doctor. There are other organizations where you may get information to help you get started. See the Appendix for more information.

You can also call your local and state medical associations for information, and they will often provide you with brochures and other print materials listing names of surgeons, as well as descriptions of certain procedures. One of the best ways to find a surgeon is by word-of-mouth. A friend or business associate may have had the most beautiful breast augmentation or face-lift you've ever seen. Obviously, these are great sources for recommending doctors. Of course, if you're absolutely certain that the lady in the next office had a face-lift, and you just love the way she looks, don't approach her about information on her doctor. She may be very embarrassed, angry, and you both could become instantly uncomfortable. Always let someone else bring up the fact that they've had plastic surgery to avoid any bad feelings, and once they do open up, then have all your questions ready.

Deciding which doctor to call can take weeks, or it can take a few minutes. However long it takes you, your next step will be making an appointment for a consultation. Just keep in mind that whoever you decide to see does not necessarily have to be the final choice. You may feel uncomfortable talking to a particular doctor, and right at home with another. One of your first clues can be showing a plastic surgeon the extra fat on your stomach and thighs, only to have the doctor mention all the other procedures that you "definitely need to have done." Some doctors may be overly anxious to redo the entire patient, and if this makes you uncomfortable, then you need to move on to another doctor.

Most plastic surgeons charge a fee for the consultation (an average cost is $50 to $100), and this could determine how many doctors you plan to see. The following section thoroughly covers the all-important consultation, hopefully answering all of your questions. You're getting closer to your goals now, and making that initial appointment will bring you that much closer.

THE FIRST MOVE: THE CONSULTATION

When you've chosen your doctor and made an appointment for the initial consultation, you'll want to be prepared with a list of questions for the surgeon. You may have read every brochure, pamphlet, and library book you could find about a procedure, but you may still be somewhat uneasy if nothing you've read has given you the facts about everything the doctor will do and how you will feel afterward. There are also many patients who *don't* want to know all the details about the procedure.

This is an important meeting for you and your doctor; have a notebook ready with every question that you may have. This is also the time to ask questions about the doctor, including education, experience, and specialties. Often, the surgeon will have an album of before-and-after photos of procedures he or she performed upon patients. This is usually a good way to see the first-hand work of the doctor and can also be an easier way for the surgeon to explain certain procedures.

You have a right to know absolutely everything the doctor will do to you, and the surgeon has an obligation to discuss your goals and expectations, as well as any possible risks and complications.

Following are some sample questions to ask the plastic surgeon at the consultation:

You: Are you in good standing with your state's licensing board?

Doctor: Yes. Would you like to see my certificate?

You: How long have you been practicing plastic surgery, and are you board certified?

Doctor: I have been practicing for more than eight years, and I have been board certified by passing oral and written exams with the American Board of Plastic and Reconstructive Surgeons.

You: What procedures do you perform most frequently?

Doctor: I have performed a full range of procedures, but the most common surgeries have been face-lifts, rhinoplasties, liposuction, and a variety of breast procedures such as augmentation, reconstruction, and reduction.

You: Do you perform surgery in your office suite, and what types of surgeries are performed there?

Doctor: Yes. I have my own surgical suite where I perform a variety of procedures, including eye surgery, laser resurfacing, and some nose surgery. Surgery requiring a general anesthetic is done in the hospital.

You: In which hospitals and surgery centers are you permitted to perform surgery?

Doctor: I can do procedures in my own office surgical suite, at Marin General Hospital, Novato Community Hospital, California Pacific Medical Center, and the Sutter Street Surgery Center.

You: Do you perform the whole surgery, or do you have an assistant help you?

Doctor: I usually do the entire surgery myself. However, in some instances, it's necessary to have another doctor assist me when several procedures are done at one time, such as reconstruction immediately following a mastectomy.

You: Who will administer the anesthesia, and what types are necessary?

Doctor: If the surgery requires only a local anesthetic, I will administer it myself. If a general anesthetic is used for more complicated procedures, an anesthesiologist will take care of this.

You: Do you teach or give lectures about plastic surgery?

Doctor: Yes. I give talks to local organizations and to the public. I also give seminars on various procedures such as laser resurfacing.

You: Have you written any books or articles about your specialty?

Doctor: Yes. I have written a book about everything a prospective patient would need to know about this type of surgery. I also publish a quarterly newsletter.

You: Can you give the names of some former patients that I can contact for references?

Doctor: Yes. After receiving permission from these patients, I would be happy to have patients contact you with your permission.

You: Do you conform to all the guidelines for sterilization and infection control of OSHA (Occupational Safety and Health Association)?

Doctor: Yes. It is of the utmost importance that these guidelines be followed to ensure total safety for the patient. We are checked regularly by this organization.

Now that you've asked these very important questions, it's time to get some answers about how this will really affect *you,* and not just a group of statistics. Here are a few more questions you might want to ask:

You: Am I ready for this surgery, or should I wait a few years?

Doctor: If you're not completely comfortable with doing it now, perhaps waiting a while would be prudent. This is not a spur-of-the-moment decision, and there are a lot of personal factors involved.

You: How long will the results last?

Doctor: That depends on the procedure and the physical shape you're in. Some face-lifts need to be re-done in three to four years, while others last much longer. Breast augmentation and reconstruction are procedures that do not usually need to be repeated. Your individual muscle tone has a lot to do with your results as well.

You: Will I have scars? Where will they be? Will they fade with time?

Doctor: Some scars remain, but they do fade with time. Scars from a face-lift are usually hidden in the hair, while those from a tummy tuck are much more visible and will remain, but will soften with time. Laser resurfacing can help.

You: How painful will the whole experience be?

Doctor: This varies with each patient and each procedure. After liposuction, some patients complain of lots of pain while most only feel sore. There is usually minimal pain after eye surgery or a face-lift. Patients undergoing breast augmentation or abdominoplasty will be uncomfortable for the first three to seven days.

You: Will I need to have someone take care of me afterward?

Doctor: After any procedure, it is necessary to at least have someone get you home and settled. With the more complicated procedures, it is a good idea to arrange for someone to care for you, your children, meals, etc., since it is necessary for you to rest and not make any sharp, sudden moves and, in some cases, raise your arms or bend over.

You: When can I go back to work?

Doctor: This depends upon the procedure. After a face-lift or nose or eye surgery, there may be some bruising and swelling for a few weeks. Plan on at least two weeks away from your workplace, sometimes less. After liposuction or eyelid surgery you may feel comfortable returning after four or five days.

You: How much is all of this going to cost?

Doctor: The fees depend upon the procedure, the facility, and the doctor's fees. (Refer to Table 3-1 for some average costs of procedures across the country.)

You: What can go wrong?

Doctor: It's very important to follow doctor's instructions both before and after your surgery. If you move too quickly, sutures can come loose. If you smoke right away, there can be complications. If you raise your arms and lift objects right after an augmentation, you're at risk for developing more swelling, and this can lead to other problems.

The initial consultation with the plastic surgeon can be a very informative experience. You've taken the trouble to make the appointment, have probably rearranged your schedule, organized rides for the kids, and have driven to the doctor's office—all in the hopes of meeting a person who can possibly help you become more self-confident and attractive.

This is usually a relaxed meeting between the patient and doctor, a time when you are literally "checking each other out." The surgeon will be considering you, your physical condition, and your expectations to see if you are, indeed, a good candidate for surgery. You, on the other hand, will be analyzing the doctor to see if you feel comfortable with him or her and to determine if professional medical knowledge, experience, and compatibility are present.

Be prepared to ask questions about details of any procedures you may be contemplating, and never feel foolish asking about the doctor's qualifications and licenses.

The consultation, which is usually your first meeting with the surgeon, includes a discussion about your medical history. Be sure to tell the doctor about any illnesses you have had (or now have), any medications you are currently taking, any to which you may be allergic, and historically, any medications or procedures you've had in the past. Often, a doctor may decide against it because it would present too high of a risk due to past problems. A complete medical examination will be done at another date during your preop appointment.

The consultation usually lasts about thirty minutes, but the amount of time will vary, depending upon the length of your discussions with the doctor and the doctor's schedule. Most doctors charge a fee for this appointment (usually about $50), but often the consultation is complementary. It is a good investment on your part because it is the best opportunity you may have to help you decide if you and the doctor have the same goals, if you are medically a good candidate for the procedure, and if you both feel comfortable.

After your visit with the doctor, the patient coordinator will compile a surgical cost analysis that is either mailed to your home after the visit or explained to you after the doctor has finished with your consultation. It will include the total fees for the surgeon's services for performing the surgery, as well as the estimated hospital fees, surgery center costs, or the fees for the doctor's in-office surgical suite. The fees involved are usually for the operation, the hospital stay (if needed), the anesthesiologist's services, anesthesia, and any medications used, and additionally, the fees of any assistant surgeons, blood donation, and laboratory and X ray services. There are often other costs, depending upon the procedure done, such as the cost of implants for breast augmentation patients and postoperative garments for liposuction patients. Many patients appreciate this information mailed to them rather than discussed in the office. This presents the opportunity to read and analyze the fees and the procedure at home and not feel any pressure.

After your consultation, you will either decide that you want to postpone your decision or will call the doctor's office to make your appointment for surgery. If, in your mind, you know that you want the surgery and its benefits, and you feel comfortable with the plastic surgeon, you have made your decision, and it's time to call the doctor's office to set a date for your preop appointment and to schedule your surgery.

From the M.D.'s Point of View: Choosing the Perfect Plastic Surgery Patient

While you're busy checking out your surgeon, he is busy checking you out as well. In his mind he is thinking, do you fit the criteria as a healthy patient, emotionally as well as physically? Will you do well after surgery? Are you a good candidate in the sense that your expectations are realistic?

A very famous plastic surgeon in San Francisco, Dr. Mark Gorney, has spent years studying patients, their expectations and goals, as well as the surgeon's goals and expectations. He teaches plastic surgeons how to choose their patients. The doctor, too, must make a decision about whether or not to operate on a particular patient.

First of all, if the patient's entire family is shaking their collective fingers about upcoming plastic surgery, and the patient has little support for proceeding, we are taught to be careful. Most surgeons will be reluctant to proceed quickly with any surgery if this is going on within the family. Again, remember that plastic surgery is purely elective surgery. During the consultation, we try to gain insight into the patient's support system and their expectations.

The Indecisive Patient

If the patient can't decide, we call them "indecisive patients." They are reluctant to make a decision. They want the doctor to make the decision for them. Some patients will ask me, "Well, what do you think, doctor? What do you think I should have?" And I will explain in detail the operations that I feel would help, but ultimately, it is their own decision, one that they will have to live with. Sometimes, I will flatly refuse to operate and state very clearly that I do not feel they are ready for plastic surgery.

The Addictive Patient

Some plastic surgery patients become addicted. They appreciate the benefits that plastic surgery has offered them. They are actually some of the best plastic surgery patients because they know they will look better afterward. But, we often look out for the extremely obsessive/compulsive patients with the "blueprints" and movie star photographs requesting the "ultimate, perfect" whatever. I am cautious with these patients, painting the picture of improvement, not perfection. Surgeons will sometimes use computer imagery to depict before-and-after shots, simulating surgery. It is important that potential surgical patients realize that the "after" picture produced by the computer may show unrealistic expectations.

Some patients are "immature" in thinking that "life" will be perfect afterward, and the girl next door will fall in love with my new nose or my new whatever. We are cautious when a patient says that her Mom wants her to have this, her boyfriend wants her to have that. As I've said before, forget it. Sometimes surgeons will know by instinct what does and doesn't work with patients.

The next chapter will deal with the various locations where your surgery may be performed—the hospital, surgery center, or the doctor's in-office surgical suite.

CHAPTER 4

WHERE SHOULD I HAVE MY SURGERY?

Once you have made the decision to have plastic surgery, you should discuss your options about the surgical location with your doctor. She will help you make the correct choice as to where you should go. You will also need to think about who will drive you and bring you home, who will take care of the children or your office, and other responsibilities that will be yours during this recovery time. You may want to have your surgery done as close to home as possible (at a surgery center or hospital) or you may want to distance yourself from the turmoil of home life; some people choose a surgeon in another state or country, close to a relative who can take care of them post-operatively while everyone thinks that they're off on some two-week dream vacation.

THE PROS AND CONS OF DOCTOR'S OFFICE FACILITIES VERSUS HOSPITALS VERSUS DAY SURGERY CENTERS

In the past, cosmetic surgery was performed only in hospitals or medical centers. Now, surgery centers—where patients can be operated on as outpatients and released the same day (for less cost)—are becoming more popular with patients.

Also, many doctors have their own surgical suites in their offices for procedures that do not require general anesthesia, and thereby eliminating the extra costs of both the surgery center and the hospital. We'll describe each of these facilities to make it easier for you to decide where to go for your procedure

THE HOSPITAL

Some plastic surgery procedures automatically require a patient to stay in the hospital for a minimum of one night. In these cases, the doctor will perform surgery in a hospital or medical center. Examples of such procedures include abdominoplasty or "tummy tuck," a thigh or buttock lift, and some cases of breast reduction.

If you are going to stay at a hospital, there is a long list of services and equipment that will be charged to you. You will be surprised to see that every move you make seems to be recorded by some invisible billing ghost that lingers somewhere in your room. Here is a sample of some of the charges you will be billed for your stay at a hospital:

- room charge
- operating room time
- medications
- intravenous solutions
- dressings
- lab work
- anesthesia and equipment

Separate charges will be billed to you by each physician involved in your surgery, including your own surgeon, the anesthesiologist, the radiologist, and the pathologist, who might study any changes in your tissue during the surgery. (Radiologists and pathologists are not usually required for cosmetic cases, however.)

In cases of normal surgery (those procedures that are medically required), most of these charges are covered by health insurance carriers. However, insurance will not cover most cases of elective surgery. As we have already discussed in Chapter 3, there are some instances when the surgery is considered "medical" in nature, or medically necessary, so it is a good idea to check with your doctor first and then your insurance carrier.

It's important to remember that you will most likely be paying the plastic surgeon in full prior to your surgery. A hospital, on the other hand, will usually require a deposit from those patients whose insurance companies do not cover the surgery.

If you decide to have your surgery at a hospital you will receive a pre-admission packet. This will include general information for patients and explains the important pre-admission appointment at the hospital, information on hospital charges, insurance, and deposit requirements. You will also receive a patient instruction sheet with further information about the pre-admission appointment, things to remember on the day of your surgery, advice on what clothing to wear, a reminder to leave valuables at home, and to make a list of any medications you are currently taking. The hospital requires that a responsible driver must take you to the hospital and drive you home afterward. Also, the hospital requests copies of your lab work results.

Patients are usually asked to call the hospital within seventy-two hours before the surgery to schedule the pre-admission appointment. At this appointment, you will pre-register, have any lab work done, receive further preop instructions, review your health history, and answer any questions.

There are advantages and disadvantages to choosing the hospital for your surgery. If your type of surgery requires an overnight stay then, of course, you don't have a choice of other options. So, if you need to be admitted for at least one night, you might as well take advantage of it.

A hospital stay can be pleasant, but it will not necessarily be serene. If you have a major procedure such as a tummy tuck, you will probably experience some discomfort as the anesthesia wears off. Therefore, you may not care about the TV, the remote control, the lonely bathroom, and the food.

One of the great disadvantages of a hospital stay is the lack of privacy. A registered nurse will visit you every few hours to check your vital signs, straighten your blanket, plump your pillows, and, essentially, not leave you alone. As soon as you close your eyes and feel relaxation setting in, it will happen all over again.

A hospital stay is also the most expensive of the three facilities to have surgery. An average price for the operating room at a hospital is approximately $1,200.00 for a two-hour blepharoplasty (upper and lower eyelid surgery). Whereas in a surgery center, the operating room fee is approximately $900.00; while the average fee for the in-office surgical suite is $600.00 to $850.00 for the same amount of time (see Tables 3-2 and 3-3 for fee schedules).

So, you can see that a hospital can be as much as three times the price of a doctor's in-office surgical suite. You may not have the luxury of choosing where to have surgery, but, when you do, we want you to be aware of the advantages of the other, more economical facilities.

THE SURGERY CENTER

The surgery center is also called an ambulatory, or outpatient, surgical center. It is a facility that offers the equipment and fully-trained staff of doctors, nurses, and technicians who perform various procedures on a same-day basis. More and more patients are choosing the surgery center for several reasons. First, the cost is well below that of most hospitals, both for the patient and the insurance companies. Second, these centers usually provide a pleasant, more intimate atmosphere in which to relax and feel comfortable. Finally, a smaller, more private facility is more conducive to visits from family and friends. In a hospital a patient will often share a room with someone else, and this can restrict private conversations with visitors.

If you decide to use a surgery center, you won't have to pay the cost of an overnight hospital stay, which can be astronomical. For instance, a patient who stays in a San Francisco hospital for a medically necessary operation such as an appendectomy will pay a minimum rate of $919.00 per day. Plastic surgery patients, on the other hand, usually pay the much lower rate of approximately $250.00 to $450.00 per day as part of a "package charge" offered by the surgeon and the hospital. These fees include costs for your room, food, and the hospital staff. So, you can actually cut the cost of your surgery by as much as 50 percent depending upon which procedure you are having done when you decide on a surgery center.

Usually, you are asked to pay one basic charge for the surgery center. This charge will include:

- medical history (or examination)
- any necessary laboratory tests
- equipment used for your procedure

- most of the supplies used
- any drugs administered to you
- anesthesia
- recovery room expenses

However, the fee for the surgery center usually does not cover:

- your doctor's professional fees
- any assistant surgeon's fees
- the anesthesiologist
- radiologist (if needed)
- pathologist (if needed)

Make sure that you check with your doctor to see if he or she has operating privileges at a surgical center in your area. If you decide that, economically, the center is the only way you'll be able to have your surgery, and if your chosen doctor can only operate in a hospital, then perhaps you should seek the services of another plastic surgeon who can offer you the advantages of a surgery center.

THE IN-OFFICE SURGICAL SUITE

The third option you might have for your operation is an in-office surgical suite. Some doctors are now performing surgeries in their own accredited operating rooms located in their offices. Not all surgeons have or need their own suite, but if your doctor can offer you this choice for your procedure, it can be a very positive experience, both financially and emotionally.

The main advantages to an in-office suite are the reduced cost, complete privacy, and a staff trained in and committed to the care of only plastic surgery patients. We have already mentioned how the office suite fees are considerably less than those of the hospital and the surgery center, but make sure you get a quote from your physician, as each doctor varies in his fee schedules. On the whole, the in-office suite is your best choice economically. However, you must make sure that your doctor can indeed perform your selected surgery in his suite, since some procedures must be performed in a hospital.

When you arrive at your plastic surgeon's office on the day of your surgery, you have probably already taken a mild sedative, such as Halcion, at home, approximately one hour before the scheduled appointment. So, when you arrive at the office, hang up your coat, and settle in with a magazine on a comfortable couch. Often, when a patient is scheduled for an in-office procedure, the doctor's staff will not schedule any other patients to be in the waiting area at the same time. Every comfort is considered to provide complete relaxation for the patient.

Once you start to feel a little groggy, you will be taken into a room where an assistant will help you undress, put on a gown, and store your purse and other belongings. You will then be taken to the surgical suite and helped onto the operating table. Unfortunately, rooms where surgery is performed are usually kept much cooler than other rooms in the office since the operating room lights increase the room's temperature. So, at first, you might feel a chill, but this will quickly pass when you are bundled up by the doctor's assistant.

Some plastic surgeon's use anesthesiologists or registered nurses to provide sedation. They will give you medication intravenously, or if called for, orally.

Having your procedure done in the office suite is actually the most comfortable, personal, and intimate way to have surgery. Another advantage is the fact that after surgery you can remain in the suite until you are ready to be driven home.

Now that we have described the different places where you can elect to have your surgery, you and your doctor need to make a decision about which facility to use. Once you've made your appointment for surgery, the next step is the all-important preop appointment, normally scheduled seven to ten days before your procedure. Chapter 5 discusses what happens next.

THE PREOP APPOINTMENT

After your initial consultation with the doctor, much soul-searching, many glances in a full-length mirror, and making the decision to go ahead with the surgery, at this point, you will need to call the patient coordinator at your surgeon's office to make all the arrangements.

The first step is to decide when you'd like the surgery performed. The date will depend, of course, on the doctor's availability and your personal schedule. Also, many patients prefer an early morning surgery so that they can wake up in the morning, go directly to the hospital, surgery center, or the doctor's surgical suite and not have to spend a long time feeling anxious about the procedure.

Next, you will need to decide where you would like to have your surgery performed—a hospital, a surgery center, or in the doctor's in-office surgical suite. We have already discussed these choices in the previous chapter, and have explained the differences of each of the types of facilities.

After the patient coordinator has checked the surgeon's schedule and has made the appointment for your surgery, she will verify the availability of the surgical location you have requested. When this has been confirmed, you are ready to come back to the office for your preop appointment.

This appointment will last approximately thirty minutes, depending upon the patient, the procedure, and any special circumstances the doctor needs to address. For instance, if you come down with a cold, the doctor will examine you and then possibly postpone your surgery.

The doctor will then explain your procedure in detail, as well as the type of anesthesia that will be used. With a general anesthesia, you will sleep through the entire operation. This type of anesthesia is normally used for procedures such as liposuction, tummy tucks, breast reduction, and other major surgeries. With a local anesthesia, only the area to be operated on is numb. This includes surgery on the upper eyelids or nose. The choice depends upon what type of surgery you are having, your doctor's opinion, and your personal feelings. Remember to have all your questions about anesthesia ready for your doctor.

The doctor will provide instructions for the night before surgery. Usually, you can have nothing to eat or drink after midnight on the night before your scheduled procedure. You may brush your teeth in the morning, but you'll be instructed not to swallow any liquid. Undigested food in the stomach can cause complications, and your surgery is likely to be postponed if you forget. Also, it is recommended that you refrain from smoking for at least two weeks before your surgery and for two weeks afterward. Some doctors also recommend taking extra doses of vitamin C for two weeks prior to surgery, as this vitamin has been helpful in fighting infections. (Nutrition is discussed further in this chapter.)

You will probably have more questions about your procedure since you last saw the doctor, and this appointment is the time to get those questions answered. There is no question that you cannot ask when the subject is your body or your face. Any doctor should be happy to answer anything you should ask.

The doctor will perform a complete medical history and physical examination, check your heart, lungs, vital signs, and review any past or present illnesses or problems. Once again, be certain to mention any medications you are taking, any allergies, and all general health problems you have experienced.

After the doctor has completed the examination, she will probably say that it's time for the "before" photographs. After any photo work is completed, the doctor's patient coordinator will enter the examination room to discuss the documents that require your signature: the general surgical consent form and the financial agreement form. The first document reflects that you recognize and completely understand the nature and consequences of your procedure(s). By signing this, the patient agrees that the doctor has explained the procedure and the risks and complications that may occur.

The second document, the financial agreement asks that you understand and certify with your signature that: "The practice of medicine is not an exact science, fees paid are for the performance of the procedure(s) only and not a guaranteed result. Although a good outcome is expected and effort has been made to establish realistic expectations, there cannot be any warranty, expressed or implied, as to the results that may be obtained. Problems relating to or complications of your surgery may result in additional costs to you. These costs may include additional anesthesia and facility fees, hospital costs, physician's fees, or other specified charges." Both of these documents are witnessed and considered legal and binding.

You may also be asked to sign a photography consent form. This acknowledges that photos can be taken at any time during your procedure, but only with the permission of your doctor. This includes permission to publish photos and information relating to your surgery in newsletters, books, and journals, but you will not be used by name. If you are uncomfortable about any part of the form, be sure to discuss it with the patient coordinator or the doctor before you sign the form. It is also okay to decline a photo consent.

Before your surgery can be performed, you will need to have some lab work done. This is ordered by your doctor's patient coordinator and is usually scheduled two to three days before your surgery date. You will receive the lab work information and order sheet at your preop appointment. Normally, the doctor will probably order four tests: a CBC (complete blood count), a UA (urinalysis), a PT (prothrombin time, to check for blood coagulation), and a PTT (partial thromboplastin time, to check for blood coagulation and clotting). You will go to a lab or the hospital for these tests. Also, if the doctor feels it is necessary, he will order an EKG to check the heart and X rays to check the lungs and chest.

NUTRITION

Another area that the doctor or his assistant will discuss with you is the importance of good nutrition in the weeks prior to surgery. Once you've decided to have the procedure, there are certain steps you should take to ensure that your body has a lot of nutritional reserves. In other words, to ensure proper healing and tissue repair, your body needs to get all the protein, calories, vitamins, and minerals that it can. The nutrients in food can strengthen your immune system and, therefore, can help prevent postoperative infection.

Adequate protein is needed to form new skin cells to cover the surgical wound and, with calories, help white blood cells function properly and help to fight bacteria. Protein is found in foods like meat, poultry, fish, eggs, beans, and nuts. Calories are also needed to ensure that several repairing processes occur.

Vitamins and minerals are also important in both repairing tissue and helping to give you a high resistance to infection. Some of the most important vitamins are C and A, zinc and iron. Foods rich in vitamin C are citrus fruit, tomatoes, bell peppers, potatoes, cabbage, and broccoli.

Vitamin A can be increased by eating such foods as milk, egg yolks, and liver. A nutrient that the body converts to vitamin A is beta carotene, and this can be found in such foods as orange-yellow and dark green vegetables and fruits such as sweet potatoes, winter squash, carrots, apricots, cantaloupe, and spinach.

Vitamin E may be recommended for two weeks after surgery, since this particular vitamin aids in healing. Often, if a patient is low in potassium, the doctor will recommend extra amounts of this element presurgery. With some liposuction patients, iron may be recommended before surgery.

Good sources of zinc include oysters, wheat germ, beans, beef, and milk; while iron can be found in foods like liver, red meat, poultry, beans, prunes, and iron-fortified cereals and breads.

If you haven't been eating a healthy variety of foods, it's a good idea to begin a new nutritional program to ensure that your body is ready for surgery. The United States Department of Agriculture recommends these daily guidelines:

> 2–3 servings — from the milk, yogurt, and cheese group
> 3–5 servings — from the vegetable group
> 6–11 servings — from breads, cereals, rice, and pastas
> 2–3 servings — of meat, poultry, fish, beans, eggs
> 2–4 servings — from the fruit group

Besides eating properly, remember to use fats, oils, and sweets sparingly, drink lots of water, and get plenty of rest.

Table 5-1.
Aspirin-Containing Products

All patients anticipating surgery MUST stop the use of all sources of aspirin or any other drugs which interfere with the blood clotting mechanism. Aspirin is a very strong anticoagulant which causes profound bleeding problems in normal individuals. Therefore, patients must stop taking aspirin and all aspirin-containing products for two weeks BEFORE surgery and two weeks AFTER surgery.

The following are only a few of many medications to be avoided:

Alka-Seltzer	Coricidin	Pepto Bismol
Anacin	Darvon Compound	Percodan
A.P.C.	Dristan	Pabirin Buffered Tabs
Ascodeen-30	Duragesic	Panalgesic
Ascriptin	Ecotrin	Persistin
Aspirin	Emprazil	Robaxisal
Aspirin Suppositories	Empirin	Sine-Aid
Bayer Aspirin	Equagesic	Sine-Off
BC Powders	Excedrin	SK-65 Compound Capsules
Buff-a-Comp	Fiorinal	Stendin
Buffadyne	Indocin	Stero-Darvon with A.S.A.
Bufferin	Measurin	Supac
Butalbital	Midol	Synalgos Capsules
Cama-Inlay Tabs	Monacet with Codeine	Synalgos D.C.
Cheracol Capsules	Motrin/Ibuprofen/Advil	Tolectin
Congespirin	Naprosyn	Triaminicin
Cope	Norgesic	Vanquish
		Zomax

If you must take something for headache, menstrual cramps, or other aches and pains, you may take Tylenol (as directed) for the two weeks prior to and after your surgery.

Source: Plastic Surgery Osler Review Course

WHAT MEDICAL PROBLEMS WILL EXCLUDE YOU AS A CANDIDATE FOR SURGERY?

First and foremost, you must be in excellent health. If your health is marginal for whatever reason, it's important to share this with your plastic surgeon. She will want to know what medications you are on; what medical problems you have; what medical problems you have had in the past, such as heart disease, lung disease, cancer, high blood pressure, and any bleeding tendencies.

I tell all my patients to discontinue all aspirin-containing products at least ten to fourteen days prior to the procedure. Table 5-1 is a list of all aspirin-containing products that affect the bleeding and can affect the overall plastic surgery operation.

Platelets are small cells in the bloodstream that help in the clotting mechanism. Unfortunately, aspirin-containing products coat these cells with a fluid that prevents the formation of a clot. If this happens, your plastic surgeon will have a difficult time controlling any bleeding. Remember, this is elective surgery, surgery you do not really need. You and your surgeon do not want anything to go wrong with this operation. She wants it to be perfect; therefore, plan on being the perfect preop patient, as well.

The following is a list of medical problems that will probably exclude you from being the perfect candidate for plastic surgery. However, there are some plastic surgeons who will opt to perform limited types of plastic surgery procedures on patients with some of these following problems:

- diabetes
- uncontrolled hypertension
- cardiac disease
- recent heart attack
- lung disease
- emphysema
- malnutrition
- psychologically unstable
- severe depression
- severely obese
- inappropriate expectations
- smoking history

Let's Talk About Smoking

Most plastic surgeons will ask their patients who smoke to discontinue three to four weeks ahead of schedule and also three to four weeks after the procedure. Some very strict guidelines are set, and patients need to stick to them. The nicotine in cigarettes or cigars causes the tiny blood vessels to constrict. The blood vessels constrict, and the skin dies and turns black, causing a horrifying condition known as skin necrosis. The same may be true of secondary smoke. (The current recommendation by most surgeons is to discontinue smoking *at least* two weeks pre and postsurgery.) The patients at greatest risk for skin necrosis are those undergoing face-lift or breast reduction, both of which depend highly upon the small blood vessels for blood supply.

If you know that you will have some difficulty quitting smoking, consult your family doctor and ask for the latest in nicotine patches, and quit. Reward yourself with plastic surgery when you do succeed. It will be well worth it.

Now that you've decided on surgery, and have had everything explained to you, it's time to pay up! Most plastic surgeons request that the patient pre-pay (in full) for any cosmetic or elective surgery at the preop appointment. So, make sure that you've brought your checkbook, credit card, cash, or money order, with you for payment at this appointment.

In approximately one week, you'll be having the surgery you've always wanted. It's about time you invested in something just for you, so everyone around you will simply have to realize that this is your time and that the necessary recovery time will require the support and understanding, not to mention help, from all of them. You now have the time to make arrangements for child-care, time off from work, have your hair done, your house cleaned, and get food stored in your freezer. Now they'll have no excuses to need you for a while, except for occasional hugs and kisses. The dog, however, might have to be trained to recognize sutures and bandages, which means "Don't jump up on the bed and lick my face!"

CHAPTER 6

CHECKING IN FOR SURGERY AND PREPARATION FOR AFTER SURGERY

It's the night before your procedure, and you're half-excited, half-nervous. You've always wanted this, and all the preparations have finally been made. But, before you go running off to your surgery, there are several important things. Please check this list to make sure you're totally prepared:

1. Do not eat or drink anything (including water) after midnight of the day preceding your surgery.
2. Bathe or shower the morning of surgery to minimize the chance of infection.
3. Absolutely do not smoke after midnight on the night before surgery. Preferably, discontinue smoking at least two weeks before surgery and two weeks after surgery.
4. Tell your doctor if you think you are pregnant since the anesthesia and any medicines may be harmful to the baby. Your doctor will give you a pregnancy test before surgery.
5. Report any health changes to your doctor such as a cough or a cold.
6. Always leave jewelry and other valuables at home.
7. Wear loose, comfortable clothing that is easy to remove and put back

on after surgery, and can stretch over large bandages and sore areas. Slip-on shoes with socks are good.

8. Bring any completed medical and insurance forms, unless you have already filled them out and turned them in.

9. Arrange for an adult to be at the hospital or surgery center with you during the surgery and to drive you home.

10. Consider filling your prescriptions before surgery.

CHECKING IN

Whenever a surgical procedure is scheduled, whether in a hospital, surgery center, or in-office suite, your presence is always requested for what seems like a lifetime before your scheduled surgery. Actually, it is much better to be early for your appointment than to hurry and risk possible delays from traffic, adding unnecessary anxiety to your already harried nerves.

You will probably be asked to arrive at the hospital approximately one to one-and-a-half hours before the scheduled appointment to ensure that all medical and insurance forms are in order, including any paperwork that wasn't completed at the pre-admissions appointment. Since there is usually no appointment like this at a surgery center, they will usually request that you check in about one hour before your appointment to take care of all the necessary paperwork. At the in-office suite, the patient who has already taken oral relaxation medication at home only needs to arrive at the scheduled surgery time. If, however, no medication was taken at home, then the patient will be asked to arrive one hour prior to the appointment, generally, but may vary depending upon your surgeon's preference.

Let's assume that you're going to have your surgery in the hospital. Your surgery is scheduled for 8:00 A.M. so plan on coming to the hospital between 6:00 and 6:30 A.M. After inquiring at the lobby information desk, the receptionist will direct you to the admitting area where you can begin your first "waiting" time until your name is called. Most waiting areas are pleasantly decorated and have plenty of magazines, bathrooms, and other pre-surgery patients.

When your name is called by an admissions representative, you'll spend about ten to fifteen minutes reviewing your paperwork. You will be asked to sign surgical permits and consent forms for the procedure that you are having done. Any unanswered questions should be asked at this point, and the plastic wristband with your name and patient number will be ceremoniously attached to your wrist.

The admitting clerk will then direct you to the day surgery department. Once there, you'll check in at the nurse's station where someone will then escort you to a room so that you can change into a gown. The nurse will then take you to a preop room where you can begin the next waiting period. This is when you will be given preop medication in the form of an injection or a pill to sedate you.

This can be a very peaceful time for the patient. You're laying on the bed thinking, I'm finally going to do this! You've probably thought about this for years, and now you are fulfilling a dream. This is a major present to yourself so lie back, relax, and let the medication take care of you.

It's probably been a long time since you've felt such peace, so enjoy every moment of it. Pretty soon, a nurse will wheel you into the operating room, which may be next door or down the hall. Either way, enjoy the ride—watch the lights on the ceiling go by, and possibly try to have some semblance of a conversation with the nurses who are "driving" you to the operating room. Once you arrive the staff will help slide you onto the table. Then, small monitors will be attached to you to monitor your blood pressure, EKG heart rate, and the oxygen in your blood.

You will have probably met your anesthesiologist on the phone the night before or in the holding area. The anesthesiologist will appear at your side in the operating room looking kind, interested, and caring. If you're having a general anesthetic, the doctor will begin administering it by first inserting an IV, a small catheter in your hand, even though the anesthesia will not be going through your body yet. The doctor will then prepare the area of your body for surgery. If you're having a face-lift, the nurses will wash the face and neck area with a special solution. So, with your plastic surgeon on one side, the anesthesiologist will be on the other. They will tell you when they are starting the anesthesia and will ask you to start counting from one hundred down. By the time you reach ninety-six or so, you will be out. And that's all there is to it!

RECOVERY PERIOD

The next thing you know, you will wake up in the recovery room, and your new nose, eyes, face, breasts, body, chin, or ears will await your viewing pleasure. But, don't look too closely or too long because the shock may be too much for you. Newly-placed stitches can be frightening at first glance, not to mention any bruising or swelling that may occur. So, while in the recovery room, try to take full advantage of this time to just lay there and relax. Nature is already starting to take its course in the healing process. One thing you might experience upon waking is the feeling that you just swallowed a cactus plant. This is due to the fact that during your surgery, the anesthesiologist inserted an LMA endotracheal tube down your throat to keep your airway open and to ensure an adequate delivery of air. The presence of this tube, which is removed before you wake up, can cause a temporary sore throat. This will subside in a short while, so don't panic and think that you picked up some virus during your procedure. You may also be very thirsty, so requesting 7 up or ice chips from the nurses will make your throat feel much better.

You may feel cold from all the time you spent in the operating room so ask for lots of blankets. It's one thing to feel like you've just been beaten up, but feeling chilled will only magnify every discomfort. You may experience some nausea, but only a small amount of patients feel sick after awakening. If this happens to you, the nurses will keep you on a liquid diet until your stomach feels calmer.

The time you spend in recovery will vary, depending upon the type of procedure you had and the type of anesthesia used. For example, an average amount of time spent after a face-lift with a general anesthetic is one to two hours. After a blepharoplasty (upper and lower eye surgery), you will be in recovery for about an hour. Abdominoplasty patients will often spend the night in the hospital, but if they are going home, they should remain in the recovery room for the maximum time allowed.

In most cases, you will feel stiff, sore, and groggy since the anesthesia will still be in effect. After you finally get dressed in your loose, comfortable clothes, and if you need any written instructions or prescriptions, you will receive them now.

If you are going home after your surgery, don't be surprised if your family goes a little crazy with their "welcome home" production. They'll probably say "How are you?" or "How do you feel?"—two totally unanswerable questions, considering you won't really know the answer to either of them.

You may have been away for a mere six hours or so, but this is still a major event in the lives of your children, your husband, wife, or friend. If you have small children, try to place them with relatives or friends for a few days so that an anxious little one won't come flying up to your lap to look at your face. It might be a good idea to have your little ones conveniently staying at a neighbor's house at the time you'll be coming home.

Your driver, who has safely gotten you home, will now have the auspicious task of getting you out of the car, into the house, down the hall, and possibly to the bathroom. The main thing to remember is to walk slowly, avoid any sharp turns and movements, and aim yourself in the direction of the bedroom or wherever you'll be spending your recovery time. It's a good idea to have your lounge outfit, pajamas, or large T-shirt, all ready and waiting on your bed. This is still your time. Let yourself recuperate. It's very important for the healing process. Before surgery, try to get as much "out of the way" as possible—errands, things to do for your children or for work, picking up some frozen foods, pizzas, and so on. Depending on your type of surgery, there are certain motions you should curtail for at least one week, if not two. For example, if you've had breast augmentation, you are not supposed to raise your arms above your head for a few weeks, so plan on having a front-opening pajama or shirt top ready when you get home.

You're just about ready to slide into the comfort of your own sheets. Someone can help you lay down, bring up your covers, and plump up your pillows. Have him adjust your windows and curtains, and put the TV remote control within easy reach. If you are hungry or thirsty, ask for whatever you'd like unless your surgeon has made specific dietary restrictions.

Make sure that your pain medication is next to your bed with plenty of water and a clock to keep track of when to take your pills. During this time, it is important for you to rest. Very few people feel like chatting, they mostly want to be left alone. There will be specific instructions postoperatively, depending on the type of operation that you've had. Reread them during your recovery. If you want solitude, don't forget to beg that you not be disturbed by anything or anyone—even the President!

There are some things you should remember during the first twenty-four hours following the procedure. Expect to be tired. You've been through a lot, both physically and emotionally, and your body needs to rest from the whole experience. If blepharoplasty (eye surgery) was performed, you will be applying ice pads to your eyes every hour for the first thirty-six hours. If you had surgery done on the head or neck, it is important that you keep your head elevated at all times, as this decreases the swelling and helps in healing. Limit your activities for the first week to relaxing, staying at home, and being totally comfortable. It's absolutely necessary that you have someone care for you during the first forty-eight hours, someone that you can count on. Friends or close relatives are often the best at helping postoperatively.

There are some downsides to your post-surgery recovery period. First of all, when the anesthetic wears off after certain procedures, you may have some discomfort. Most doctors prescribe pain pills. Ice packs and heating pads are usually not recommended postoperatively, as there is always the chance that newly-moved tissue will be bruised. There will probably be little or no pain after a face-lift, eye surgery, or breast reduction, but you will feel stiff and tight. If you do experience pain, the medication will help you feel better.

It is quite common to feel happy and elated after plastic surgery. It's all over, you're excited about your new look. This usually lasts about two to three days. Even though you may feel great, what you're feeling is a sort of euphoria or a sense of well-being and relief that the procedure is behind you. However, it is not uncommon to experience a mood swing soon after—a depression may set in or a general sense of disappointment after the initial thrill is gone. You will look in the mirror, and gaze upon a swollen and bruised stranger unable to visualize the final results. You may want to cry and not want anyone to see you. You might want to become an instant hermit, wondering if you should have had the surgery and spent the money. These thoughts are very, very common and will fade away when the swelling and the bruising improve and results become evident.

During this period you'll really need the support and understanding of your family and friends during the early postoperative weeks. So, perhaps you should warn them ahead of time that you might turn into a real monster for a while. Your surgeon will also be an important person to consult regarding questions and concerns.

You should follow your doctor's instructions after surgery. Failure to do so could result in complications or injury. Driving a car must be postponed until you are off medication and your surgeon gives you the "okay." Safe driving judgments can be affected and any movements made while driving—sharp turns, stopping short, or even colliding with something—can cause sutures to come loose, incisions to separate, and bleeding to occur which can lead to hematomas and many other problems.

Also, in the first twenty-four hours after surgery make sure that you do not sign any important papers or make any significant decisions. You should not drink any alcoholic beverages or take any medicine not prescribed by your doctor. You'll need to eat a light diet for the first twenty-four hours. As mentioned earlier, you may feel sleepy, nauseated, and lightheaded as a result of the anesthesia, and rich, heavy foods might make you feel sick.

FOLLOW-UP VISITS

Your follow-up visits to the plastic surgeon will vary depending upon the procedure you've had done and the doctor's preference. If you have had a breast reduction with a one to two day hospital stay, the doctor will come to your room and examine you twenty-four hours or so after your surgery. If you had outpatient surgery and went home to recuperate, as in the case of a breast augmentation, face-lift, and most cases of liposuction, then you'll need to have someone drive you to the office. You are not permitted to drive from four to ten days after a breast augmentation and even longer for abdominoplasty and liposuction due to any anesthesia and medication that might still be in your system and also to protect your wounds and sutures from any sharp movements or sudden stops. If, for example, you've had liposuction on a Tuesday, the doctor will probably want to examine you on Friday, again in a week, and then in two weeks. Once again, the amount of follow-up visits will be determined by your doctor.

During your follow-up, the doctor will change any dressings and bandages, examine your sutures, and check for any excessive swelling or bleeding that might have occurred, as well as signs of infection, redness, or swelling.

The follow-up visits are very important for the doctor as well as the patient. It is necessary for the physician to closely monitor the progress of the surgery and the subsequent sutures, swelling, and changes in muscle and tissue. Several things may be discussed during these visits with regard to wound care and bandages, and what to expect postoperatively regarding swelling and bruising during recovery. Your physician's office staff will be your main "reality check" when it comes to your concerns and questions about your recovery. Keep the doctor's phone number close by, and call with any concerns or questions.

Once you have healed and the swelling has dissipated, your surgeon will consider taking the "after" shots. These are usually done in the same position and lighting as the first pictures to enable you both to truly see the improvements. Some physicians have professional photographers take pictures. Please remember that each doctor has his or her own schedules and techniques for these photographs, and the procedures of one office are not necessarily the same at another.

Dealing With the Change After Plastic Surgery

It is not uncommon after plastic surgery to feel some depression, some misgivings early on. Should I have spent all of this money, or should I have just lived with what I had? It especially doesn't help the patient when family members are saying, "I can't believe you went and had plastic surgery . . . You didn't really need it."

As a plastic surgeon and also a plastic surgery patient, I know what it feels like during this recovery process. Initially, it is very difficult. You feel like you're not the same person; part of you is lost. This short period of depression usually lasts two to seven days postoperatively. However, with time, and it doesn't take much time, one gets to like the new, improved look. I can't tell you how many times I heard, "I wish I'd done it sooner. My friends all tell me I look so good. I haven't told them why. I want to keep it my secret."

Are You Ready for the New You?

Some plastic surgery procedures are easier to accept than others, such as a face-lift, eyelid procedure, breast augmentation, and tummy tuck. These procedures improve a patient's appearance yet not so dramatically that the personality of the patient has changed. When it comes to rhinoplasty, or nose, operation, the change is more difficult to accept. It is often easier to make a major change on a seventeen-year-old than it is to make a major change on a forty-five or fifty-year-old person. Psychologically, a seventeen-year-old can deal with a major change, whereas a forty-five-year-old has been looking at the same nose for the past forty-five years and will have some difficulty accepting a major change. However, minor rhinoplasties can be performed, and patients do extremely well. Rhinoplasty is still appropriate for this age range, but subtle, more refined changes are usually helpful.

Most patients, before they even have plastic surgery, ruminate about it. "Should I or shouldn't I? Oh, it's so vain. I'm not that vain that I need plastic surgery. I'm not going to tell anybody that I'm going to have it done." Ruminate, ruminate, ruminate, schedule, cancel, reschedule, etc. The majority of patients are extremely happy with plastic surgery afterward.

I do slide shows for career days at the local schools in my community. I show before-and-after pictures of patients to second, fourth, fifth, and eighth graders, and they all see the benefits and the improvements gained by plastic surgery. When I ask, "Which picture do you like better?" it's always the "after" shot that gets the vote.

With most patients, the depression lasts for a short period of time. If it persists longer than two weeks, most surgeons recommend consultation with a psychologist or a psychiatrist.

The majority of patients are ready for their "new" look. Once the swelling improves, the sutures are removed. People begin to feel a new self-confidence and self-esteem, and they begin to come out of any short-term blue period.

In our next several chapters, we will explain several plastic surgery procedures so that you will better understand what you will experience. We have found that most people are very interested in exactly what happens to them during their surgery. We hope the next chapters will answer any of your questions. Remember, if you have any questions about any of these procedures, talk to your plastic surgeon about anything that you do not understand.

CHAPTER 7

THE PROCEDURES:

A Brief Outline of Cosmetic, Surgical, and Non-Surgical Procedures

Now that we've introduced you to plastic surgery, the next chapters discuss the different types of procedures that are currently being performed by plastic surgeons in the United States as well as abroad. Some of the discussion will include commonplace plastic surgery procedures, which are the majority of plastic surgeons' work. Other discussion will include procedures that may not be common to all plastic surgeons, but can still be performed. We will also include new procedures, the "cutting edge" of plastic surgery, what we will be seeing in the year 2000 and beyond.

But first, let's go back in time for a moment. As a plastic surgeon, I often wonder if the Mona Lisa herself could be improved with plastic surgery. The Mona Lisa, as you know, is a famous painting by Leonardo da Vinci. The painting has been treasured for many years and for her famous crooked smile. My theory is that the Mona Lisa apparently developed facial paralysis, possibly from Bell's palsy, but it could have been from a long list of other possible causes. Facial paralysis occurs when the nerves that supply the muscles of the face stop working, preventing a person from smiling, blinking, and opening and closing the mouth. Usually only one side at a time is affected—giving an afflicted person a very asymmetrical smile. Well, this brings us to plastic surgery in the nineties.

Today, if Mona Lisa were to walk into a plastic surgeon's office, she'd need help. (Mind you, in the picture it is oh so slight a difference between the two sides.) However, if she were smiling just a little bit more, we might really be able to see the difference in her smile. But speaking theoretically, yes, she might have been an excellent candidate for plastic surgery.

To decide if you would be an excellent candidate, make out a list on a sheet of paper the procedure that interests you and weigh the risks and benefits of the procedure. Visit with the doctor on more than one occasion. Review the section in this book that fits with what you are considering. Ask lots of questions, and make lists of questions. Good luck on your journey.

The following chapters discuss these procedures:

- face-lift
- brow lift, temporal lift
- blepharoplasty
- neck lift
- breast surgeries, breast reductions, breast augmentations
- rhinoplasty
- liposuction
- laser surgery
- dermabrasion, collagen, and other injectables
- lip augmentation and reduction
- abdominoplasty
- arm lifts, thigh lifts, and buttock lifts
- cheek implants, chin implants, and chin reductions
- men and plastic surgery
- hair transplants
- permanent tattoo
- Retin-A and alphahydroxy acids
- what can go wrong and complications
- revisionary procedures
- other times you might need a plastic surgeon

THE LUNCH-HOUR PROCEDURES

Some patients are in such a hurry to have plastic surgery. The following is a list of some procedures which can literally be done during one's lunch hour:

1. Injection to help improve the frown lines above the nose, in the forehead, and around the eyes.
2. Collagen injections to erase the lines around the eyes, lips, and face, as well as to enhance narrow, thin lips.
3. Laser resurfacing to eliminate the wrinkles around the eyes and on your face. Vascular laser for spider veins.
4. Injection to remove spider veins in the legs. Laser of vascular lesions of the face, laser of pigmented lesions on the face and/or hands. Hair removal by laser.
5. Removal of an unsightly mole.
6. Permanent tattoo for the eyes, eyebrows, or lips, or removal of tattoo.
7. Mild revision of previous plastic surgery.
8. Minor eye lift.
9. Minor liposuction of one area or two.
10. Minor nose surgery.
11. Hair transplant surgery in a small area.

Consult the following chapters for a full discussion of the procedures.

CHAPTER 8

THE FACE-LIFT

In this chapter and in subsequent chapters, we will describe several plastic surgery procedures to help you understand what your surgeon will be doing during each individual procedure. We'll explain what happens in normal cases, but please remember that, no two cases are alike, each patient is different, and final results may vary. So, let's begin with the rhytidectomy or face-lift.

FACE-LIFT OR RHYTIDECTOMY: WHO'S A CANDIDATE?

One of the more popular procedures in plastic surgery is the face-lift. The average age range for face-lift candidates was once between sixty and seventy. Now surgeons are performing face-lifts on patients in their late thirties and forties. The baby boomers have arrived, and the over-forty crowd doesn't want the young or the very old helping out. Our patients want to look "terrific."

A face-lift cannot stop the aging process, but it can help the patient look and, therefore, feel younger. During a face-lift, or rhytidectomy, excess fat is removed, underlying muscles are tightened, the skin is repositioned or stretched back over the face and neck, and excess skin is removed.

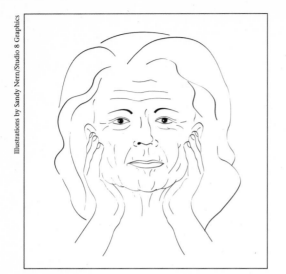 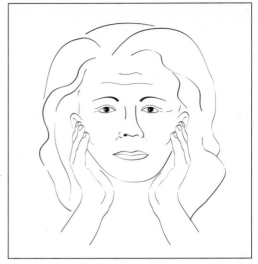

Figure 8-1. Pulling back the face with your hands can simulate what a face-lift can do for you. Removing excess skin will help eliminate wrinkles.

WHAT ARE THE DETAILS OF THE OPERATION?

Generally speaking, when a patient undergoes a face-lift, we usually recommend that this be performed under general anesthesia, or sometimes under local anesthesia with intravenous sedation. The procedure lasts anywhere from three to five hours depending on how extensive the procedure. The patient is brought into the operating room in a wheelchair or gurney and then transferred to the operating room table. Once the patient is comfortable, the anesthesiologist gives the patient some sedation through a catheter in a vein. Following this, the general anesthesia or IV medications will allow the patient to be comfortable. The doctor is now ready to start locating the position of the incisions. Usually the incisions for a face-lift procedure are right in front of the ears and right behind the ears, extending back into the scalp area. Oftentimes, the incision will be extended up along the hairline just above the ear on both sides as well, as this will help improve the wrinkles around the eye area and the temple area. In the past ten years, surgeons have commonly performed a face-lift in conjunction with a brow lift. As we age, our entire face ages, not just the lower half. Oftentimes, a brow lift (see Chapter 9) will help rejuvenate the "superior" upper half of the face where wrinkles form across the forehead and between the eyebrows. A brow lift may also be done separately, but

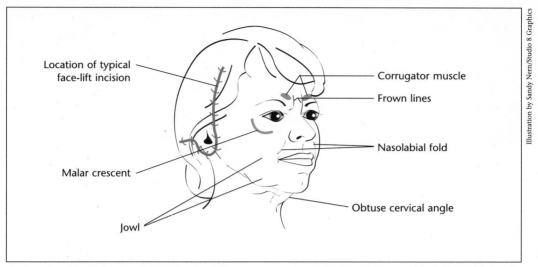

Figure 8-2. Superficial topography. These are the areas of the face that plastic surgeons concentrate on when performing a face-lift.

many patients prefer to combine it with their face-lift, thereby eliminating a separate surgery and the additional preparations and recovery that are required.

After the incisions are outlined, the patient is injected with some local anesthesia into the area of the face or the area that will be worked on. Following this, the face will be cleansed with an antiseptic soap, sterile sheets will be placed around the face, and the surgeon will begin the operation.

The skin is "elevated" or lifted off the muscles in the face in an upward direction toward the cheek area or around the neck on both sides. The skin is also raised off the forehead area if a brow lift is to be performed. Sometimes surgeons will do more extensive operations depending on the needs of the patient. For example, people who are older will generally need more extensive dissections requiring elevation of muscle and the SMAS layer. SMAS is an abbreviation for superficial musculo aponeurotic system—a superficial tissue layer that covers the muscles of the face. If a SMAS dissection is performed, the surgeon will require more time to complete the procedure, but the face-lift may also last longer.

The lower half of the face is a concern for most people in the forty to sixty to seventy to eighty age group, and the most common area worked on in a face-lift procedure. Thus, real attention is directed toward the area underneath the chin.

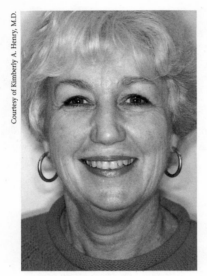

Courtesy of Kimberly A. Henry, M.D.

Figure 8-3. Before a face-lift and neck lift

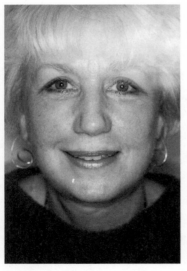

Figure 8-3. After a face-lift and neck lift

The muscles (the platysmal bands) are brought together to improve the muscle bands underneath the neck (commonly known as "turkey neck"). Fatty tissue can be removed from underneath the chin area, and, occasionally, liposuction is used in these cases. A small incision is placed just underneath the chin-line area, and fat can be suctioned out or removed directly.

Following the elevation of all the skin in the cheek and lower neck area, the skin is then lifted and pulled back. Excess skin is removed and the closure of the incision is begun. Sometimes surgeons will use staples in the hairline as this decreases the amount of hair loss, since staples swell and prevent tightness that a suture would cause. Following the closure, surgeons sometimes place drains, which will generally be kept in place for approximately twenty-four hours. These drains are thin tubes made of soft plastic that are inserted behind the ear to drain any excess fluids immediately following the procedure.

In my patients, I usually place a head wrap dressing around the areas of incisions following the procedure. This is removed in a few days along with the drains. Many people experience a minimal amount of pain following the surgery; however, they do feel a sense of tightness around the neck area, which can be present for two to three weeks but will gradually improve over the next several months. Most patients usually go home a few hours after the face-lift procedure; however, some patients opt to spend the night either in a special retreat recommended by the physician or in a hospital setting if they've had prolonged anesthesia or surgery later in the day. Most patients prefer to have their surgery performed early in the day; however, often the doctors and surgical facilities have schedules that can only permit late afternoon surgeries. In these cases, it may be recommended that you spend the night in the hospital.

Postoperatively, elevation is important. Patients must sleep with their head elevated, as this will decrease the swelling around the facial area. Some people use recliners, while others opt for six to eight pillows to prop them up in bed. Oftentimes with a face-lift procedure, people will have other procedures performed at the same time such as their upper and lower eyelids, a nasal procedure, a chin augmentation, malar (or cheek) augmentation, and, as we mentioned, a forehead lift. Please refer to the other sections for information.

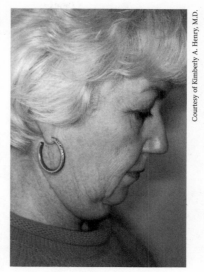

Figure 8-4. Before a face-lift and upper and lower lid blepharoplasty

Occasionally, following the procedure, there can be some concerns with regard to the healing process. It's very important that you have not ingested aspirin, Motrin, or Advil prior to the procedure at least two weeks ahead of time. Patients who ingest these types of medication can develop some bleeding problems. In addition, it's important if you have high blood pressure that you take your blood pressure medication, as this can lead to problems with bleeding and hematomas, which can occur following these procedures. The worst case scenario is when a patient calls from home and complains of some swelling around her face on one side more than another. Any time I hear this type of concern, I immediately see the patient

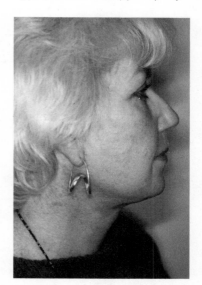

Figure 8-4. After a face-lift and upper and lower lid blepharoplasty

either in the emergency room or at my office. I release the bandage, and if there's fullness on one side, it's consistent with a hematoma, or a blood collection underneath the skin flap. This is a surgical emergency that needs to be treated, usually in an operating room. The final result is not generally affected.

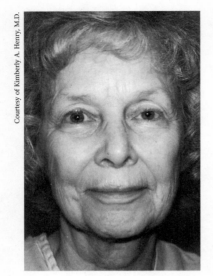

Courtesy of Kimberly A. Henry, M.D.

Figure 8-5. This woman opted for a face-lift and blepharoplasty.

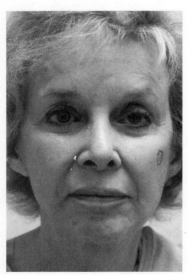

Figure 8-5. After surgery, she looks ten years younger.

As the patient is recovering, some numbness in the skin may occur, but this is normal, and it will disappear in a few weeks or months.

What Kind of Improvement Can I Expect?

After the shock of seeing a bruised and swollen face when the bandages are removed and a few deep breaths, the face-lift patient can be assured that this is the worst she will look. Every day of recovery will bring more improvement, and in a few weeks, the mirror should show a truly improved face. It's important to take it easy for the first week after surgery, avoiding strenuous activity for four to six weeks, as well as alcohol and steam baths. Outdoor sun exposure should be kept to a minimum, and remember to get plenty of rest. Soon, your beautiful new face will affect a more contented, happy outlook on life.

After any plastic surgery procedure, there will be a few patients who are not "ready" to go through the recovery phase. Oftentimes, people are ecstatic after their procedure, then within forty-eight to seventy-two hours, they become somewhat blue. "Why did I even have this done? When am I going to look better? My husband thinks it was ridiculous that I had this done." But as the swelling improves and the bruises disappear, so does their mild depression. Once fully recovered, they're very glad they had it done.

NEW TECHNIQUES IN A NUTSHELL

The new techniques of face-lifting have promising applications, but whether or not they last long remains uncertain.

- Some techniques require an incision just behind the ear for patients with problems only in the neck area. Other procedures utilize the suspension of several sutures around the neck area, similar to a purse string held taut, which creates a nice angle of the jaw.
- Laser resurfacing combined with a face-lift helps eliminate fine wrinkles not often eliminated with just a face-lift.
- Fat injections can be used to augment certain areas, giving more fullness to the cheek, lip, and chin areas.
- Augmentation with silastic implants in the cheek and chin area can also be performed with a face-lift, which improves the overall result as well.
- Some of the techniques presented by Drs. Sam Hamra and Jack Owsley incorporate cheek elevation during the face-lift which further aids in the rejuvenation of the aging face.
- Lastly, the endoscope, which is the hottest item out there, second to the laser, can also be used for the face-lift. It's main use currently is in the area of the brow lift, but some surgeons are experimenting with its use in the cheek/mid face and neck area as well.

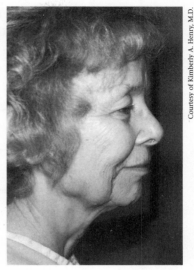

Courtesy of Kimberly A. Henry, M.D.

Figure 8-6. Before a face-lift and blepharoplasty.

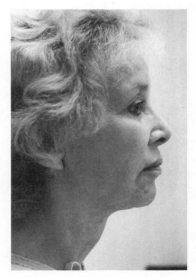

Figure 8-6. After a face-lift and blepharoplasty. Note the overall improvement.

The ultimate goal for any plastic surgeon is to perform a face-lift without using an incision, perhaps one of these days, but not soon.

Figure 8-7.
Rhytidectomy or Face-Lift

Recovery Time	Risk Factor	Pain Factor	Cost Factor
Initial: 7–10 days *Complete:* 3–4 weeks	Minimal if a patient is in excellent health	Mild discomfort	$3,000–$15,000

CHAPTER 9

THE BROW LIFT

One day after a Rotary luncheon where I had spoken about plastic surgery, a man came up to me to ask, "Can you make me look less angry and sinister looking?" He did look angry, although he was a very jovial person. His face didn't fit his personality in any way. He was the perfect candidate for a brow lift. When I examined him, he had droopy, ptotic eyebrows. Needless to say, he made an appointment, I performed the operation, and he was quite happy with his new look.

The brow lift operation is specifically designed to treat the tired, stern, angry look of the upper face. It helps treat the lines that develop across the forehead from the use of the muscles of the forehead, and it can help eliminate hooding, droopy eyebrows, forehead lines, and the frown lines that come with age. A brow lift creates a face that looks more alert and youthful.

This operation has been around for several years, but it has become increasingly popular during the past ten years. Famous plastic surgeons such as Sam Hamra and Peter McKinney have realized that a face-lift alone does not completely rejuvenate the face, and combining the two operations significantly improves a patient's overall appearance.

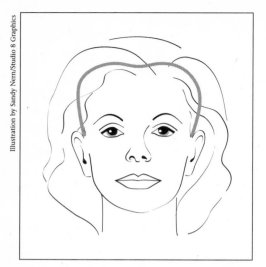

Illustration by Sandy Nern/Studio 8 Graphics

Figure 9-1. Bicoronal incision for a forehead lift

The upper third of the face ages with the lower two thirds of the face, and this operation can help balance out the aging face, especially if a face-lift is performed on the lower half. Sometimes people opt to have a face-lift but not a brow lift. The lower half of the face looks younger while the eyes and forehead look older. So when you're considering a face-lift, ask your surgeon if a brow lift also needs to be done.

If the brows descend below the orbital rims, they are said to be "ptotic" (pronounced "totic," the "p" is silent). This is what makes people look tired and angry. Take a look in the mirror, and see where your brows line up. Sometimes an eyebrow can be higher than another eyebrow, and this can also be an indication for a brow lift. Most people, when they are looking in the mirror or having a picture taken, raise their eyebrows, so a true evaluation of brow ptosis is not really evident unless the patient is holding quite still. During a consultation with a patient, I usually massage the forehead with my fingers and then let them take a peek in the mirror to see the true position of the eyebrows.

THE PROCEDURE

There are several different possibilities for incision locations, and determining which is best will require some thought. Most surgeons currently use the bicoronal approach, which is an incision about 5 to 7 centimeters behind the hairline extending from ear to ear. The greatest advantage to the bicoronal incision is that it is hidden in the hairline (see Figure 9-1). If your forehead is rather broad and long, the surgeon makes a pretrichlear incision that begins right at the hairline. Another technique involves direct brow incision just above the eyebrow. Excess skin is then excised to help reposition the eyebrow (see Figure 9-2). Other patients opt for incisions that go straight into an already existing forehead crease, which is common in men losing their hair. You and your surgeon must decide on the best incision for you. The more advanced technique of brow lift—the endoscopic approach—is discussed below.

How Long Is the Operation?

The operation can be performed under general anesthesia or under IV sedation. Most surgeons take anywhere from two to three hours to perform the procedure. He will usually close the incision in layers with a deeper subcuticular stitch, which is absorbed by the body, followed by either staples or sutures. Surgeons often opt for staples because they swell along with the tissue, inhibiting any injury to the fine hair follicles of the scalp—thus preventing hair loss along the incision.

Postoperatively, the patient can expect to be a little black and blue around the eyes. I usually dress the patient in the operating room in a "mummy wrap." They go home wearing the same bandage and return the following morning for removal. Patients are allowed to wash their hair the following day and wear it the way they normally would. Most of the swelling occurs around the eye area so I ask my patients to apply ice compresses to help decrease any purple bruising that may occur. During the recovery period, we ask the patient to keep their head elevated on three to four pillows. The recovery is similar to that of a face-lift, and you will notice a rapid improvement around your eyebrow location. You will no longer have a tired angry look. For some patients the creases of the forehead will be completely erased and for others made significantly better.

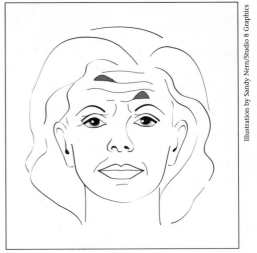

Figure 9-2. Direct excision

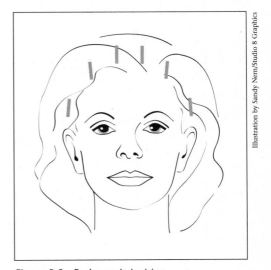

Figure 9-3. Endoscopic incision

Illustration by Sandy Nern/Studio 8 Graphics

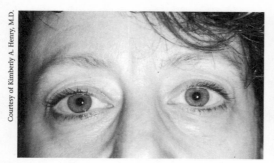

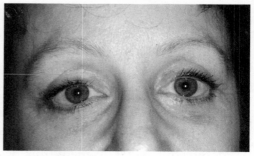

Figure 9-4. This patient was concerned about always looking mad and tired.

Figure 9-4. After a brow lift in conjunction with an upper and lower lid blepharoplasty.

Expect the skin in front of the scalp incision to be a little numb up to 3 to 4 centimeters in front of the incision. With time, the nerves will reinnervate and numbness will lessen. Sometimes patients have drains placed, which are removed on the first or second day postop.

Staples usually remain intact for about eight to ten days. Doctors watch for bleeding and infection postoperatively, both of which are quite rare. Occasionally, temporary hair loss can occur near the incisions, but this improves within four to six months. In this case, some surgeons will place micro-hair tufts along the incision, a new technique that helps eliminate any possible hair loss. Most patients return to work within one to two weeks.

THE LATEST ENDOSCOPIC BROW LIFT— A NEW SUBSTITUTE

Over the past four to five years, the endoscopic brow lift has become the latest technology in the treatment of brow ptosis, corrugator muscle hypertrophy, and frontalis muscle hypertrophy. The procedure is similar to the surgical removal of a gallbladder using an endoscope. A camera is attached to a long tube called an endoscope, and special instruments are used in the tiny incisions in the stomach/abdominal region to remove the gallbladder.

Plastic surgeons are using the same approach in the brow region to help eliminate the long bicoronal incision from "ear to ear." The endoscopic brow lift approach uses approximately five 2-centimeter incisions in the normal area where

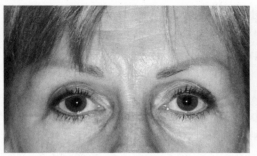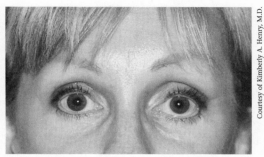

Courtesy of Kimberly A. Henry, M.D.

Figure 9-5. Notice the forehead creases and wrinkling between the eyebrows. An endoscopic brow lift improves the frown lines leaving a more serene, youthful look.

a brow lift incision would be located. The endoscope helps lift up the tissue of the forehead; the corrugator muscles (the muscles that create the frown lines between the eyebrows) are then removed with special scissors. See Figure 9-3 for endoscopic brow lift incisions.

After a brow lift, many patients tell me they are glad I recommended it to them, as they had never understood why they looked angry, sad, or tired. It has eliminated their lines of the forehead, smoothed out the skin, and created a more alert and youthful appearance. I remember having one patient who, following this procedure, said that when she got mad at her kids, they just laughed at her because she now had a much more "pleasant look" on her face.

The before-and-after pictures, Figures 9-4 and 9-5, depict the expected results following a traditional brow lift and an endoscopic brow lift.

Figure 9-6.
Brow Lift—Elevation of the Eyebrows

Recovery Time	Risk Factor	Pain Factor	Cost Factor
Initial: 3–5 days *Complete:* 10–12 weeks	Minimal if a patient is in excellent health	Minimal	*Brow lift:* $3,000–$3,300 *Endoscopic approach:* $3,500–$4,500

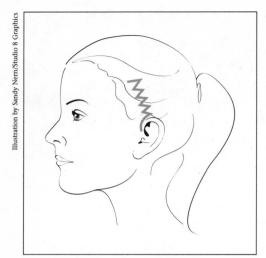

Illustration by Sandy Nern/Studio 8 Graphics

Figure 9-7. Zigzag incision for a temporal lift

The Temporal Lift— For When You're not Ready for a Full Brow Lift

Those who are not quite sure about a brow lift, but want some improvement should consider the temporal lift. Many patients may seek the services of a plastic surgeon in their mid-thirties, concerned about significant lateral brow ptosis, where the eyebrow drops off to the side near the temple area. This causes a person to look very tired, and with some minimal elevation, we are able to open up the eyes, open up the eyebrows, and have patients look much more youthful in appearance rather than sad and angry.

The procedure can be performed under direct local, IV sedation, or even general anesthesia. It is very similar to a brow lift, but the incisions are placed in the temporal area only. The temple area is infiltrated with local anesthetic, and an incision is made. The surgeon undermines the area, lifts and excises excess skin, and closes the area with sutures and staples. This helps draw the skin up from the eyebrow area, lifting the eyes to a higher level, helping the overall appearance in this area. The identical procedure is performed on the opposite side.

The benefit of a temporal lift is that the patient doesn't have a full incision needed for a brow lift. It gives distinct elevation in the area of concern. Most patients prefer this less invasive procedure, but not all patients are good candidates. Some may really need a full brow lift, and this is something that will need to be evaluated with your plastic surgeon. Reorienting them inappropriately can make a person look too surprised or, in some cases, worried. A well-trained plastic surgeon knows exactly where they should be positioned.

When patients interested in an elevation of their brows come to see me, I evaluate what really needs to be elevated—what part of the brow needs to be lifted. I usually position the patients in front of the mirror and elevate the skin to show them what they may look like with a brow lift or a temporal lift. It's important not to lift the brows too high, especially the inner brow, as this may make the person look bewildered. Some patients ask to lift them only a small amount. Others want a significant amount of lifting. Each case is very individual, and it is very important that you let your doctor know your feelings about your anticipated outcome.

Occasionally, other procedures can be incorporated with a brow lift. The most common is the eye lift or blepharoplasty. The combination of a brow lift and eye lift will result in a dramatic improvement for a patient. However, they must, of course, be candidates for the combination.

Again, it's very common after any of these forehead lifting procedures to develop some numbness around the incision. It will take some time to get better.

Some patients opt for an even less invasive procedure such as BOTOX injections to help decrease the functioning of the "worry" corrugator muscles of the forehead.

Figure 9-8.
Temporal Lift

Recovery Time	Risk Factor	Pain Factor	Cost Factor
Initial: 2–4 days *Complete:* 10 days	Minimal	Minimal	$1,500–$2,500

BOTOX INJECTIONS FOR ANGRY LINES: THE TEMPORARY SOLUTION

BOTOX (Botulinum Toxin Type A) purified neurotoxin complex is a protein produced by the bacterium *Clostridium botulinum*. The effects of the botulinum have been well known since the early 1900s, but it was first used in the medical field in the early 1980s to treat many ophthalmologic problems related to the muscles of the eyes.

Currently plastic surgeons use the toxin to treat creases formed by the two horizontal muscles of the forehead which are located between the eyebrows (the corrugator muscles). Many people are told that they look mad or angry, when in fact it is just the deep creases formed by these muscles.

The botulinum toxin can be injected into these muscles causing them to "go to sleep" for a period of up to six months. Most patients see nice results for up to four months following the injection.

When I had my first BOTOX injection I could see immediate results the first day, and by the end of the week I could not wrinkle or make a mean face. My face was much smoother and much more relaxed. My office manager, who also had the injection, said she felt like her skin had been smoothed out or stretched, resulting in a much more serene look.

How Does It Work?

The toxin of BOTOX is a nerve impulse blocker. It binds to the nerve endings and blocks the release of chemical transmitters that activate muscles. The transmitter chemicals carry the "message" from the brain that causes a muscle to contract; if the message is blocked by the BOTOX injection, the muscle won't work.

It is important to realize that BOTOX injections are not permanent. It is an effective temporary treatment, but you will probably require repeat injections. However, it can be the preliminary step to the more involved brow lifts that can permanently remove the corrugator muscles and stretch out the lines created by the function of these muscles.

Occasionally, patients do not opt for the brow lift because they are either concerned about the incision or just not quite ready yet. I will often recommend BOTOX injections initially so that patients develop an understanding of what a brow lift can do for the hyperfunctioning muscles of the forehead. The BOTOX injection temporarily obliterates the function of the corrugator muscle, which is the main small muscle on both sides of the nose just above and between the eyebrows. The BOTOX injection lasts three to four months.

Figure 9-9.
BOTOX Injection

Recovery Time	Risk Factor	Pain Factor	Cost Factor
Immediate	Minimal	Short-lived headache 3–4 hours after injection	$500–$750/ injection

CHAPTER 10

THE BLEPHAROPLASTY, OR EYELID PROCEDURE:

The Most Common Operation Performed

Blepharoplasty is the term for the plastic surgery procedures that correct aging of the eyelids. Many surgeons feel that eyelid surgery helps a person look more alert, attentive, and fresher than any other surgical procedure they do. The eyes are the main point people fix on when looking at someone's face, the "pathway to the soul." If they are hidden by excess skin, wrinkles, and puffy deposits of fat and muscle, they are not attractive or happy and sometimes they are mean and tired looking. Interestingly, of all the plastic surgery procedures that men opt to have, this is the most common. And, most men do it for business reasons, to remain competitive in the job market or at work.

WILL MY FACE LOOK BETTER BY JUST HAVING MY EYES DONE?

The blepharoplasty will make a person appear less tired and more youthful. Most people seeking blepharoplasty will usually require both upper and lower eyelid procedures. However, some patients are not convinced that they need both and opt for having the upper or lower done individually. Some people don't necessarily need

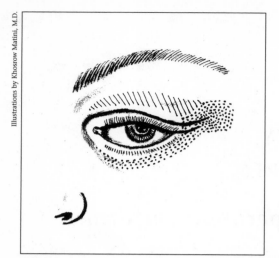
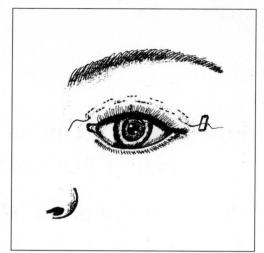

Figure 10-1. Before and after upper and lower lid blepharoplasty. Excess skin is excised from the upper lid, and excess fat is removed from the lower lid.

both, but this is rare. Individually, the upper eyelids usually need to be done if a person has a lot of excess upper eyelid skin redundancy. Sometimes it is so excessive in older people that the skin actually inhibits vision. We call this loss of the peripheral visual fields and an ophthalmologist will document this. If loss of vision is significant, an ophthalmologist will recommend an upper lid blepharoplasty, and in this case, a patient will be covered under their insurance policy for this type of procedure.

UPPER LID BLEPHAROPLASTY

The operation will be performed either in a doctor's setting or hospital setting. The operation takes approximately one hour to one hour fifteen minutes. The excess skin is outlined, and the skin is injected with local anesthetic. Sometimes an anesthesiologist will be present to administer medication to make you drowsy for the procedure.

Excess skin is excised, and the redundant two pockets of fat are removed. Following this, the sutures are placed and remain in place for four to five days until removal by your surgeon. Once the sutures are removed, makeup may be applied usually, but consult with your surgeon. Expect to look black and blue during the

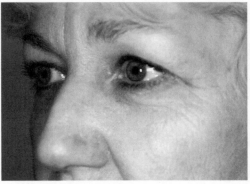
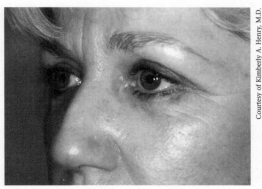

Figure 10-2. Before and after upper and lower lid blepharoplasty. The plastic surgeon concentrates on removing droopy eye lid skin and puffy lower lid fat during an eye lift.

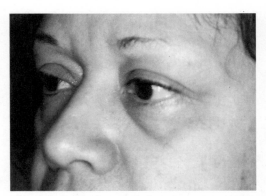
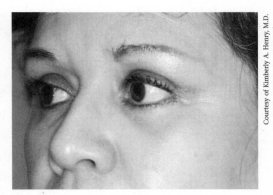

Figure 10-3. Blepharoplasty improves upper and lower lid puffiness.

first seventy-two hours. This may last anywhere from five to ten days. Most patients take off work for about seven days.

LOWER LID BLEPHAROPLASTY

Lower lid blepharoplasty removes excess fat which has "herniated" through the soft tissues surrounding the globes. This helps eliminate what we call "the bags" of the lower eyelids. The bags really make us look tired. During this operation, an incision is made just below the eyelashes. Excess fat is removed. (There are three small fat pads.) The puffier the eyes, the larger the fat pads. Excess skin and muscle is redraped. Crow's feet can be touched up with the laser or chemical peel four to six weeks after the operation, but sometimes surgeons will do it at the same time depending upon the location of the incisions. Most patients return to work soon after the sutures are removed.

Expect to have puffy eyes for about two weeks postoperatively. You may have the continual feeling of dry eyes for a few months until your eyes adjust. We usually recommend eyedrops continuously every two to three hours during this time.

POSTOPERATIVE: WHAT CAN I EXPECT?

The first forty-eight hours should be spent taking it relatively easy. It's important that you sleep with your head elevated. I have my patients place four-by-four inch iced gauze on their eyes. Some surgeons use small balloons filled with frozen peas. All of this will really help with the swelling and bruising that will normally occur with any patient.

GETTING USED TO THE NEW LOOK

Every week and every month that goes by will help you get more and more used to your new look. You will like it better and better as time goes on. Initially, people are concerned about looking tired; with time, this will improve. Your eyes will begin to look more elegant, sophisticated, and less "tired looking."

In the next chapter, we will be concentrating on the neck area, along with liposuction.

Figure 10-4.
Blepharoplasty—Eyelids

Recovery Factor	Risk Factor	Pain Factor	Cost Factor
Initial: Black and blue around eyes for 7 days. Some patients may have small areas of residual bruising. *Complete:* 10 days	Minimal if a patient is in excellent health	Minimal when compared to other operations	$1,700 or $3,000–$4,000 *(upper/lower lids)*

CHAPTER 11

THE NECK LIFT

I often have patients come to see me who are in their late twenties and late thirties who have a significant amount of fatty tissue below their neck region. It's not that they're aging quickly over time or that they are overweight, it's just that people often have a genetic predisposition to developing an "obtuse neck," one with a significant amount of fat and very little definition in the jaw (mandibular) border. Everyone in the family usually has it.

Liposuction alone can help improve some of the problems in the area of the neck. But oftentimes, if a person would like strong definition and the most improvement, liposuction plus a face-lift or neck lift helps improve the overall appearance. Adding a chin implant in some appropriate cases helps the overall result significantly. Sometimes the submandibular salivary glands need to be removed. The combination procedure of liposuction with the neck lift or face-lift will immediately improve the appearance of the patient with an obtuse-angle neck, creating more definition of the angle of the jaw.

In addition, many patients express concern about wrinkles around the neck, what I call "necklace wrinkles." A neck lift or face-lift will help this. At this point, the Ultra Pulse CO_2 laser is being utilized to treat wrinkles of the face, and it can be used in conjunction with a face-lift. The laser is only being used on an experimental basis for wrinkles of the neck area. Perhaps we will be using it in the future to replace face-lifts, but at this point, it is only used after a face-lift has been performed to treat wrinkles not improved by a face-lift.

THE NECK: DO I NEED A FACE-LIFT OR LIPOSUCTION?

Below you will see an outline of diagrams of necks in profile. Generally speaking, most patients that see me about the neck area are in their early forties to mid-seventies, but some are younger, as mentioned earlier. Following is a list of "neck deformities" and treatment possibilities:

Deformity #1: Excess fat and youthful skin in a young patient. The treatment is liposuction only with a twenty-four-hour use of a fitted garment of the neck area to give support for at least fourteen days.

Deformity #2: Excess fat and excess skin. Liposuction, direct excision of fatty tissue as well as a face-lift is needed to help improve the contour of the neck area. Both fat and skin have to be removed in order to improve the overall contour.

Deformity #3: Congenital or acquired retrognathia, the term used to describe a small chin. The treatment is chin implant if not severe; otherwise oral maxillofacial surgery will be required to reposition the bony tissue of the jaw line.

Deformity #4: Some patients have no excess fat but a significant amount of excessive skin. The treatment for this is a face-lift or a mini-neck lift.

Whatever your situation is, your plastic surgeon will discuss in detail the differences and the combinations and what would be best for you before proceeding with an operation.

Sometimes during the face-lift, your surgeon will opt to reposition and work with the platysmal muscle of the neck. This is the main muscle of the neck, and when repositioned appropriately, it will give a wonderful contour to the neck region. This is considered a part of the SMAS face-lift procedure. The platysmal muscle plays

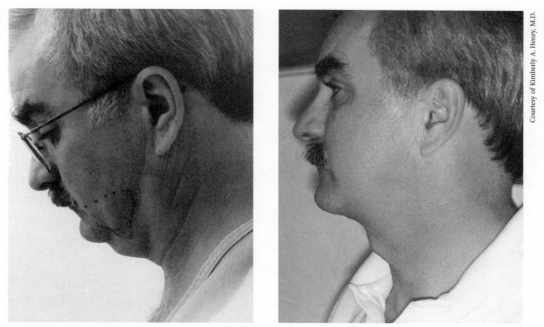

Courtesy of Kimberly A. Henry, M.D.

Figure 11-1. The man featured in this picture underwent liposuction of the neck area as well as a small tuck underneath the chin area.

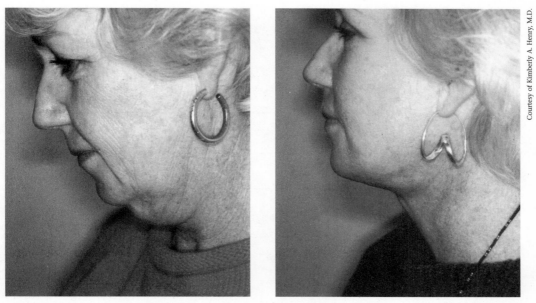

Courtesy of Kimberly A. Henry, M.D.

Figure 11-2. This woman underwent liposuction in combination with a neck lift because of excessive skin and fatty tissue underneath the chin.

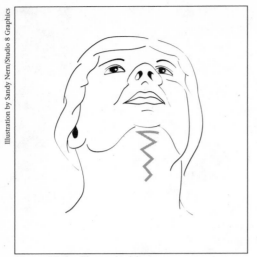

Illustration by Sandy Nern/Studio 8 Graphics

Figure 11-3. Zigzag incision

a large part in the creation of the "turkey" neck that people often refer to.

I usually reserve this for men in their fifties, sixties, and seventies, making an incision in the skin of the neck and directly excising excess skin which can lead to a beautiful result. The diagram of the procedure is shown in Figure 11-3.

The Z-plasty or zigzag incision heals very nicely. The incision cannot be made as a straight line in the neck area, otherwise the patient would develop a severe scar contracture, causing the chin to slowly move down toward the chest wall. The multiple Zs displace the formation of scar tissue creating a proper balance in scar contracture. Most men are very happy with the final result. It is especially effective for the older patient who may not be healthy enough for a full face-lift or for those who prefer a less invasive procedure than the full neck lift. Patients who have high blood pressure or who are not interested in having incisions around other areas will also benefit from this type of procedure.

Figure 11-4.
Neck Lift

Recovery Factor	Risk Factor	Pain Factor	Cost Factor
Liposuction— *Initial:* 3–5 days *Complete:* 10 days	Minimal if a patient is in good health	Mild	$1,500–$4,500
Neck lift— *Initial:* 7 days *Complete:* 14 days	Minimal if a patient is in good health	Mild to Moderate	$3,000–$15,000

CHAPTER 12

BREAST AUGMENTATION

B reast augmentation, or augmentation mammoplasty, has become one of the most requested plastic surgery procedures by women of all ages. It is performed for several reasons, most commonly, to increase the size of small breasts; correct a difference in size between the breasts; and for breast reconstruction following mastectomy for breast cancer. A breast implant is inserted either behind the breast tissue of each breast or behind the pectoralis major muscle, the major muscle of the chest wall, thereby increasing the size of the breast.

Breast augmentation has been around since 1962, and both saline and silicone implants have been available to women since then, up until 1992. At that point, the Federal Drug Administration (FDA) set a moratorium on silicone gel implants preventing the use of these type of implants for breast augmentation. Currently, there are two companies in the United States making breast implants, Mentor and McGhan. Currently, Mentor is the only one associated with the FDA and has a formal study program to evaluate breast implants. In May of 1995, Mentor provided a quick response information service in Santa Barbara, California, which revealed seventeen major United States and international studies that have consistently shown no link between implants and disease.

In addition, the British government has reviewed the research on implants and has determined no evidence of an increased risk of connective tissue disease and, therefore, no scientific case for changing the policy and practice in the United Kingdom. The French government recently lifted its ban on gel implants after reviewing this same research. Although silicone is used in a wide variety of life-saving devices and technologies, lawsuits from silicone breast implant patients threaten its availability.

The implants currently on the market are more durable than the ones first developed in 1962. The actual capsule itself is thicker and made of solid silicone; the inside of the implant is empty and is usually filled with saline or an antibiotic solution at the time of surgery.

Gel implants remain available to patients, but they must be part of an FDA-Mentor study and must satisfy specific criteria to be in the study.

As a practicing plastic surgeon, my thoughts regarding implants are mixed. Should we leave the breast implants in place or recommend that they be removed? Who knows? I have removed implants from patients with autoimmune disease, and their autoimmune disease improved. For others, there was no change.

Dr. Joan Campagna, a well-known rheumatologist, is conducting a considerable amount of research in this area of implants. We are all busy awaiting her recommendations. She currently recommends the placement of saline implants for those interested in breast augmentation.

It is true that many medical devices such as heart valves, catheters, and cataract lenses contain Silastic/silicone and do not cause problems to other types of medical patients.

AUGMENTATION FOR SMALL BREASTS

The most common reason for breast augmentation is to increase the size of small breasts. Patients are either born with small breasts or they develop a loss of some breast tissue following breast-feeding, pregnancy, or weight loss. The procedure is relatively easy to perform, and many of these procedures are done each year here in the United States and around the world. (See Figures 12-1 to 12-3.)

The Doctor's Company, a prominent malpractice insurance carrier, has prepared a document which outlines a comprehensive checklist for patients and their

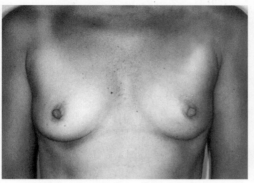
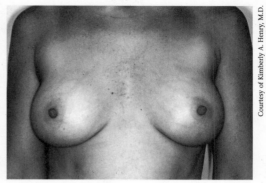

Courtesy of Kimberly A. Henry, M.D.

Figure 12-1. This woman had lost some fullness in her breasts after breast-feeding two children. She opted for breast augmentation with saline implants.

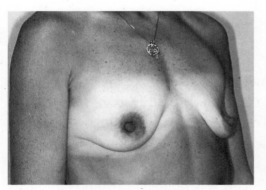
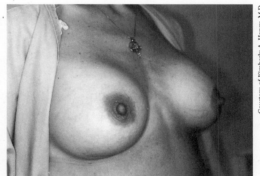

Courtesy of Kimberly A. Henry, M.D.

FIGURE 12-2. This mother of four opted for augmentation with saline implants after having breast-fed four children.

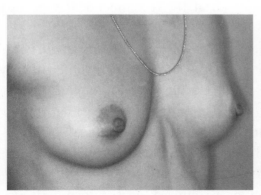
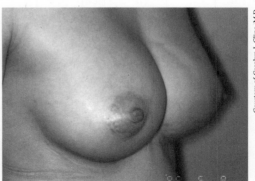

Courtesy of Carolyn J. Cline, M.D.

Figure 12-3. Before and after breast augmentation with saline implants placed in the submuscular position.

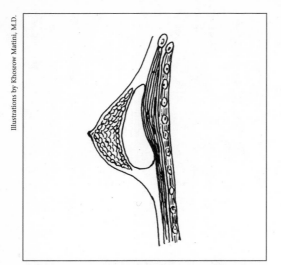

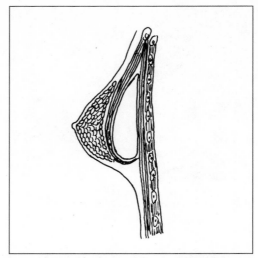

Figure 12-4. Submammary implant. The implant is placed just underneath breast tissue.

Figure 12-5. Submuscular implant. The majority of implants are placed below the pectoralis major muscle.

plastic surgeons to review and discuss prior to the procedure. Whenever I see a patient for breast augmentation, I review this form. In consultation, I first discuss alternative operative procedures. Some techniques of fat transfer have been suggested in the past but are currently not recommended as fat grafts can create "calcifications" preventing accurate mammographic analysis for breast cancer.

Each plastic surgeon has their own specific way of doing the procedure. This procedure is usually performed under general anesthesia, but it can be done under IV sedation as well. Most surgeons using saline implants have been placing the saline implants underneath the pectoralis major at the recommendation of the implant companies.

As for the anticipated outcome and anticipated size, it's important that patients bring pictures to the consultation. The idea of "beauty" is different for everybody. The average size of a woman who has undergone breast augmentation is approximately a "C" cup. Some women will opt for a "D" or larger, but this is something that needs to be discussed with your plastic surgeon ahead of time. Sometimes, there are constraints on an individual's anatomy, in which case, a woman who is very small and petite would not tolerate a "D" or "DD." The implants would be too large to insert. The most common breast implants size is anywhere from 270 to 375 ccs of normal saline.

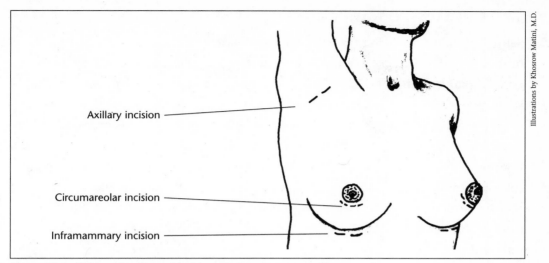

Illustrations by Khosrow Matini, M.D.

Figure 12-6. Different locations of incisions for breast augmentation

ONE BREAST IS LARGER THAN THE OTHER

If asymmetry, or a difference in size between the two breasts, exists, a complete correction is unlikely, but breast augmentation using two different sizes can help. Asymmetry exists in all patients. Sometimes it's a subtle difference, other times the volume difference is quite obvious. Your plastic surgeon can help correct the difference with implants of different sizes.

LOCATION OF INCISIONS

The most common incision made is an *inframammary* approach which is an incision just underneath the fold of the breast. Another approach is in the *circumareolar* area, an incision just around the lower part of the areola (the darker area of the nipple; while the third approach is in the underarm or *axilla* area. All incisions heal relatively well. Your surgeon will discuss the appropriate incision for you. Some surgeons are able to use a special endoscope and place breast implants through a small incision in the belly-button (umbilicus). However, very few surgeons are currently trained in this technique.

TYPES OF IMPLANTS AVAILABLE

Saline implants are currently available to all women interested in breast augmentation. If patients who have previously undergone breast augmentation with silicone implants wish to have silicone implants again, they will be made available to these patients, but they are required to become part of an ongoing FDA-Mentor study. Occasionally, a woman who has had saline implants and is bothered by any problems or concerns with them, has the option to switch over to silicone depending upon whether or not she satisfies the criteria for the Mentor study: thin skin, severe wrinkling, ptosis, or for breast reconstruction. If a patient has undergone a breast augmentation with saline implants and is unhappy with the "feel" of the implant, they may satisfy criteria of the FDA-Mentor study to have silicone implants placed instead. Plastic surgeons must satisfy special requirements with the FDA-Mentor and their local hospital investigation review board before they're allowed to place silicone implants.

The Saline Breast Implant Versus the Silicone Breast Implant

The advantages and disadvantages of saline and silicone implants are always included during my pre-operative consultation:

Saline Implants: Advantages and Disadvantages

- No known connection with autoimmune disease.
- If it ruptures, your body will absorb the saline fluid.
- Occasionally, patients will feel the side of the implant, a "rippling" of the implant. If the implant is under just breast tissue, you may actually see "rippling." A surgeon must overfill the implant by 10 percent to eliminate some of the rippling.
- The feel of the implant may be firm, whereas silicone implants feel more like breast tissue.
- Safe per the FDA's current recommendation.
- Recommended by most rheumatologists as an alternative to silicone augmentation.
- Less incidence of capsulary contracture (scarring around the implant).

Silicone Implants: Advantages and Disadvantages

- Concern for connection with autoimmune diseases.
- If it ruptures, the body will not absorb the silicone.
- Silicone has been found in the local and distant lymph nodes and may travel to other locations and affect us systemically—how it does, at this point, nobody knows.
- Feels more like breast tissue.
- Increased incidence of capsular-scarring contracture.

INHERENT RISKS INVOLVED

The main goal of this procedure and all procedures is to have satisfied patients who are happy and ecstatic about their results. However, as with any operation, there are some inherent risks involved, the main three being bleeding, infection, and scarring, specifically related to the implant capsular contraction formation (scarring around the implant).

Every single person who undergoes augmentation will have a foreign body reaction to the implant. The degree to which this occurs depends upon your own individual response and how you heal. Some people develop so much scar tissue that the implants become quite firm. A classification system called Baker's class I, II, III, and IV has been used to classify the severity of the reaction.

Baker's class I shows no scar contracture. Class II and class III are differing degrees of scar contracture. Class IV results in significant, painful, noticeable contraction. If a contracture does occur, it can be improved with placement of the implant under the muscle or switching over to saline implants. When the implant is replaced and/or the scar tissue removed, it is only necessary to use the same incision. The final healing of the incision will probably be no different than before. Currently, there's a smooth-walled implant as well as a textured-wall implant. This textured-wall implant tends to decrease the amount of capsulary contracture around the implant because it disorients the collagen bundles.

Ruptured Implants: What Happens, What Can I Do?
There is always a possibility for future rupture of your implants. The older the implant, the more likely it is to rupture. If a patient is involved in a ski accident,

hits the steering wheel hard, is assaulted, or the breast implant receives a strong blow, there is a strong possibility that the implant will rupture. A routine mammogram can also rupture an implant. If an implant does rupture, one of the following may happen: If it is saline, the breast implant will go flat as a pancake, and the body automatically absorbs the saline. Some patients develop a fever and rash with the rupture of a saline implant. If it's a silicone implant, the rupture is harder to detect. The breast may lose it's overall shape. There may be distortion or an irregular shape. Sometimes a doctor needs to order a mammogram to detect the rupture of an implant, or an MRI, the more specific test, to determine if an implant is ruptured. If an implant is twelve to thirteen years old, it is most likely ruptured, and most surgeons recommend removal. Often, if the implants have been in place for this length of time, patients opt for replacement with a newer type of implant.

The most important risk for any breast augmentation patient is the possible decreased ability to detect breast cancer in the future. I recommend to most of my patients who undergo breast augmentation to have the breast implant placed underneath the muscle. This helps to improve the detection of breast cancer if they develop a breast mass and actually improves the ability to see the breast tissue following a mammogram. Another view, called an Ecklund view, helps aid the further detection of breast cancer.

There are other rare and unsubstantiated, but possible, relationships to connective tissue disorders such as rheumatoid arthritis, lupus, and scleroderma.

Future Pregnancy and Nursing

There are many patients with breast augmentation who have successfully been able to breast-feed their children. The operation itself does not affect the milk ducts, so architecturally the operation is theoretically safe. If a patient is interested in breast-feeding after augmentation, there should not be any difficulty. However, some women are not able to breast-feed no matter what, and it has nothing to do with the breast implants.

Complications

Complications are always a possibility, as with any operation, although they are rare. The main ones in this case are infection, bleeding, excess or obvious scars, or changes in nipple sensation. With regard to infection, it's very important that the plastic surgeon place you on antibiotics both during and after the procedure. It's important that you take every single antibiotic and not miss any. The implant is a foreign body that is being placed into your body under sterile conditions, but if you are prone to infection, you may develop one. If an infection does occur, your surgeon has to be notified right away. Signs of infection include redness, tenderness, drainage from the wound, fever, and chills.

Infection

If an infection cannot be improved with oral antibiotics, IV antibiotics administered by a catheter into your vein need to begin right away. If the infection does not improve with the antibiotics, the plastic surgeon may recommend removal of the breast implants as a temporary measure, replacing them three months later. Patients who are poor candidates for breast implants and more likely to develop infection are those with diabetes, those who have problems with poor wound healing, or those with compromised immune systems, such as patients with kidney transplants, asthma, those taking the medication Prednisone, or those who have the AIDS virus.

Bleeding Postoperatively

Bleeding is very rare, but it can occur with this operation. It's important that patients discontinue the ingestion of aspirin, Motrin, Advil, Alka-Seltzer, or any aspirin-containing products prior to surgery. Aspirin affects the clotting factors and platelets in the blood which control the bleeding. Bleeding will present as increased swelling on one side or the other. A patient should call their plastic surgeon immediately if they notice fullness on the breast wall on either side. If this happens, it is necessary to take the patient back to the operating room and remove any kind of fluid or blood collection (hematoma). The implant is left in place, and the incision is closed. There should be no problem with the final result unless the hematoma is not caught early enough or treated appropriately.

Scarring

The excess or obvious scar depends upon the patient's wound-healing ability and genetics. Different techniques can improve the scarring. For instance, for hypopigmented or very pale white scars, the plastic surgeon may recommend tattooing

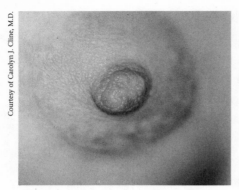

FIGURE 12-7. Postoperative periareolar scar.

around the nipple areolar complex or around the suture line. Often with the raised scars, we can inject them with steroids, vitamin E, or Silastic sheeting. Chronic pain is rare, but it can occur. Ninety-nine percent of patients who have breast implants are extremely happy with them.

As far as the expense of breast augmentation, the fees depend on the location in the nation. It's more expensive in New York than in Colorado or Nebraska. However, the implants themselves are usually the same price across the nation. The implants range anywhere from $1,000 a pair for saline to $1,800 a pair for silicone.

Occasionally, revisions need to be done. Implants may need to be changed for larger or smaller ones, and most surgeons will do this at a reduced fee, but this needs to be discussed ahead of time.

BREAST IMPLANT REMOVAL AND AUTOIMMUNE DISEASE

Frequently, people come to see me for breast implant removal. Oftentimes, they are self-referred because of the implant scare or are sent to me by rheumatologists who feel that the implants should be removed. I have removed breast implants on some women who have been very concerned with having the implants in place. The actual procedure of removing the implants is relatively easy. The implant is removed through the same incision and the capsule around the implant is removed in its entirety. If there is any rupture of the silicone, it is important to remove the entire capsule as the silicone particles can be embedded into tissue surrounding the area. This is more technically involved, but most board certified plastic surgeons can surgically perform a total capsulectomy.

The implants, if they are silicone, can be replaced with saline. Many patients who have had previous silicone implants and are concerned about the possible but currently unsubstantiated autoimmune problems will often switch to saline implants. The saline makes the patients feel much more safe, making treatment more comfortable. A few patients who have had the implants removed opt not to replace them. Some of these patients do quite well, while others experience some difficulty accepting the fact that they no longer have the fullness they had with the breast augmentation. Sometimes this loss is very similar to a woman who has undergone a bilateral mastectomy, and there can be significant depression that needs to be worked through. I had one patient who had breast reconstruction and then decided to have her breast implants removed following the procedure. She was concerned about any effect the implants would have on her autoimmune system, and although she was depressed initially, she eventually re-channeled her energies into her business and family which helped her through the crisis period.

RECOVERY

During postoperative recovery, you will be limited in your activities. This means no rigorous aerobic classes or dancing for approximately four to six weeks. Mothers of small children should not pick them up. Have someone place them in your lap while sitting on a couch or on the floor. I often recommend that my patients not take up skydiving, skiing, or aggressive tackle football. If, for any reason, there is a significant amount of pressure directed to the implant, the implant could rupture.

After a breast augmentation, the patient will probably feel tired and sore, but bedrest and medication will help the discomfort level. Within two to three days, most women are walking and performing normal daily activities. It is very important, once again, not to lift anything heavy and to wear a bra as directed by your physician, as your breasts will probably be sensitive. Sutures are removed in ten to fourteen days; scars will remain pink for at least six months, sometimes longer; and the swelling may take three to four months to completely disappear.

Augmentation patients are usually ecstatic about the results of their surgery, and they almost always feel better about themselves.

THE FUTURE IMPLANT

At this point, the main implant available to patients is the saline implant. In the future, and perhaps sooner than the next five years, Trilucent breast implants, sugar implants, and possibly soybean oil implants may become available. Trial studies are currently being done to evaluate the trilucent implant which will allow a mammogram to see completely through the implant. At any rate, implant companies are quickly looking into providing patients with the ultimate implant that is both safe and feels as much like normal breast tissue as possible.

Almost all implants, both saline and silicone and possibly the newer experimental implants are currently available in Europe and Canada. South America is also providing women with the controversial silicone implants at this time.

Figure 12–8.
Breast Augmentation

Recovery Time	Risk Factor	Pain Factor	Cost Factor
Initial: 4 days *Complete:* 2–3 weeks	Minimal if the patient is in good health	Moderate— Most patients are uncomfortable for the first 4 days	*Saline implants:* $1,300 *Silicone implants:* $1,800 *Surgeon's fees:* $2,500–$4,000

CHAPTER 13

BREAST REDUCTION

Another common procedure performed in plastic surgery, and one that produces patients who are extremely happy with the results, is breast reduction. Often, a woman who has breasts that are very large experiences both physical and emotional discomfort. These women are excellent candidates for breast reduction surgery. Women with naturally large breasts can be bothered with severe neck pain, back pain, shoulder strap tenderness, indentations from the bra straps, and the psychological effects of having very large breasts. Girls who develop large breasts at a young age are often teased and can become the object of jokes. Breast reduction can help these women, both physically and emotionally.

Breast reduction has been available for many years, and the procedure is becoming more and more refined. The most common type of breast reduction is the McKissick breast reduction. This procedure involves removing breast tissue from the right and left sides of each breast and repositioning the nipple which remains attached to breast tissue throughout the procedure. At the end, a patient will have an incision around the nipple areolar complex and underneath the breast. (See Figure 13-1.)

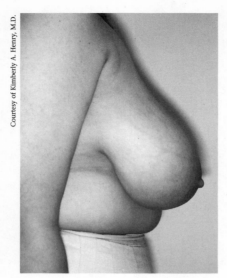

Figure 13-1. Before breast reduction, the patient was a size 38DD and complained of severe back and neck problems.

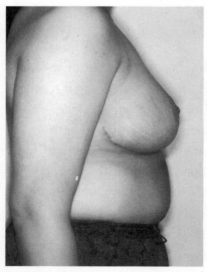

Figure 13-1. After breast reduction, she is now down to a size 38C and much more comfortable.

Prior to this operation, it is *very* important that a patient not smoke, as there can be some problems with poor wound healing and poor blood supply to the nipple areolar complex. A patient who does smoke needs to stop at least two weeks ahead of time and for at least two weeks after the surgery.

WILL MY INSURANCE COVER THIS?

Often, this procedure is covered by insurance companies, and after a consultation, the surgeon will obtain pictures and send them to the insurance company with a letter for pre-authorization for the procedure. If the patient is significantly debilitated as a result of large breasts, the plastic surgeon will express those concerns when presenting the case to the carrier. Although some insurance companies are becoming more strict about authorizing breast reduction, it is usually medically necessary for the well-being of the patient. Often, the company asks the patient to lose weight or to attend physical therapy sessions prior to authorizing the surgery.

Once a breast reduction is authorized by an insurance company, the goals and expectations of both patient and doctor are discussed in detail. One of the main concerns for the patient will be the acceptance of the scar that normally results from this procedure. Most women are so happy about the improvement in their body contour as well as the decrease of neck and back pain, they could care less about the incisions. I hear satisfaction and relief from these women, rather than concerns about the scars.

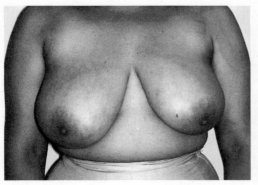

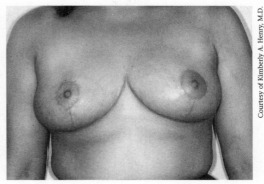

Courtesy of Kimberly A. Henry, M.D.

Figure 13-2. Breast assymetry is common to many women.

Figure 13-2. Breast reduction improves the symmetry and size. These incisions are typical to breast reduction procedures.

THE PROCEDURE

I usually have my patients check into the hospital the morning of the surgery, usually between 6:00 and 6:30 A.M., as these surgeries are often scheduled at 8:00 A.M. I meet them in the holding area before the operation and draw some markings on the breasts with a purple surgical marking pen which is permanent during the surgery, as well as postoperatively for a few days but will quickly fade.

Symmetry is an important aspect of this procedure. Oftentimes, my patients will have asymmetry between the two sides with one breast being larger than the other. If the left breast is a bit larger than the right, this is taken into consideration, and the procedure is modified appropriately. The nipples will be repositioned. The normal nipple position from the point at the base of the neck is anywhere from 19 to 23 centimeters, depending upon the height of the patient. If breasts are ptotic, or droopy, the nipple has to be repositioned to a higher point. These markings done before the operation are probably the most important part of the entire operation. If the markings are done correctly then the patient will have beautiful results.

Following this, we bring the patient into the operating room, place her on the operating table, and the anesthesiologist administers general anesthesia. During the operation, the patient is positioned symmetrically on the operating room table. Oftentimes, I will use a second plastic surgeon to assist during the operation in order to save time on anesthesia and to allow for improved symmetry between the right and left breasts. We usually operate simultaneously, using two teams of nurses to help us with the procedure.

Following the breast reduction, the incisions are closed with sutures. I usually use sutures that are buried underneath the skin and dissolve on their own, although I will occasionally use some sutures that have to be removed in one to two weeks following the procedure. Most patients prefer sutures that dissolve and leave very few stitch marks. This type of closure is called a subcuticular closure. In addition, with every breast reduction that I do, I use drains which are removed the following day. Some plastic surgeons opt not to use drains, but this decision depends on their experience and personal preference. I also use a breast wrap which consists of a Kerlex roll, a gauze roll that looks like a mummy wrap around the breast area and is changed daily for about two weeks. Each surgeon has his or her own preferences for postsurgery dressing, some using gauze and some suggesting the use of a bra immediately after surgery. We recommend avoiding an underwire, as this can cause more irritation to the incision line. We also recommend a bra that is supportive, especially in the area on the outside, near the arm, as the breast tissue will continue to mold and form for the next four to six months. The final result of the shape of the breast is not evident for up to six to eight months postoperatively. Following the surgery, the incisions will be red and noticeable for up to one year.

COMPLICATIONS

The main complications from this kind of procedure are bleeding and infection. On occasion, one of the patient's breasts might become more swollen than the other. This is a sign of a hematoma, a fluid collection, or bleeding. If this occurs, it is necessary to take the patient back to the operating room where general anesthesia is once again administered. The previous incisions are re-opened, and any hematoma can be evacuated and bleeding controlled. The incisions are re-closed, and in most cases, the patient's healing process should progress normally.

A second concern is infection. The patient is covered with intravenous antibiotics before, during, and after the procedure to allow as much protection as possible. Breast infections are uncommon, but if they do occur, it's very important that your plastic surgeon begin IV antibiotics or oral antibiotics immediately. Signs of infection include redness, tenderness, fever or chills, or purulent drainage coming from the incision line.

At about four to six weeks the incisions look the best that they will look. At about eight to ten weeks they start looking quite red and noticeable and lumpy and bumpy. Do not despair. There are some things that your plastic surgeon can recommend such as applying vitamin E oil to the incision line. Break a small capsule with a sterile pin and allow the capsule to drain onto the incision line and rub the vitamin E oil into the incision line. In addition, a new technique using Silastic sheeting, which has been around for approximately four or five years, helps compress the scar and will help minimize the final scar. If you have significant scarring, the third option is steroid injections. The only problem with this option is that occasionally it can cause widening of the scar. However, small amounts of steroid injection are often appropriate and can really help the improvement of scars.

Most patients, immediately after the procedure, feel a significant improvement in their back pain/neck pain. They no longer have the feeling of "heaviness." After a breast reduction patients will often look at their stomach and say, "Oh my goodness, I could never see my stomach like this before!" Sometimes patients undergoing breast reduction are also candidates for an abdominoplasty, or tummy tuck. Occasionally, we sometimes combine the two procedures with patients who are in excellent health. This occasionally requires an extra night in the hospital as opposed to staying only one night or going home the day of the procedure. When an abdominoplasty—a major procedure in itself—is combined with a breast reduction, it is important that the patient be monitored closely and that the hospital staff is readily available for the comfort of the patient.

Following instructions about ambulation or movement following the procedure is extremely crucial. Patients must limit activity for four to six weeks and no heavy lifting must be attempted. If the patient has small children, it is important that she not lift them but, rather, relegate this duty to someone else. If a patient is young and considering this procedure, we sometimes recommend postponing the surgery (unless the breasts are quite large) until after childbirth. However, there are some patients who are so large by the age of fifteen or so that a breast reduction is indicated to prevent further back problems.

After the surgery, the patient may feel some discomfort for a few days when moving or walking, but medication and rest will aid in this recovery. Bandages or dressings will be removed a day or two after surgery, but it is necessary to wear the surgical bra continually for several weeks until the swelling and bruising have dissipated. Stitches are removed in one to three weeks. It is not unusual to experience sharp pains in the breast area, a loss of sensation in the nipples, and general soreness, but this will greatly improve with time. The patient can usually return to work in about two to four weeks.

Oftentimes, it is necessary to perform two and three breast reductions on patients. I remember one patient who was about eighteen or nineteen and ready to go off to college. We performed a breast reduction, and she returned a year later requiring another breast reduction because her breasts continued to grow following the surgery. There may be continued growth of the breasts, and in these cases, a breast reduction can intervene only temporarily. It's very important that the patient understand that, although rare, there is always a possibility for repeating the breast reduction again in the future.

DETECTING BREAST CANCER
DURING A BREAST REDUCTION

For patients over the age of thirty-five to forty with a family history of breast cancer, it's *really* important to obtain a preoperative mammogram that can often detect early signs of breast cancer. The increased incidence of breast cancer in our nation makes it important to keep track of this, especially if somebody is going to undergo surgery. A breast exam is extremely important before any type of breast surgery as well. In approximately 7 percent of patients undergoing breast reduction, we can spot breast cancers during the breast reduction procedure. The specimen, as in all cases, is sent for pathologic examination to be evaluated by a pathologist. If breast cancer is indicated, a mastectomy *will not* be done in the operating room at the time you are undergoing breast reduction.

If breast cancer is suspected or found, your plastic surgeon will consult with you following the procedure. She will let you know that some suspicious tissue was found during the breast reduction, that it was evaluated by the pathologist, and it was found to be breast cancer. The plastic surgeon will then recommend consultation with a general surgeon, and other options of breast surgery will be discussed in detail.

THE LATEST TECHNIQUES

There are other techniques currently being presented for breast reduction. These include liposuction, as well as two techniques developed by European surgeons Lejour and Benelli, which call for smaller incisions. Dr. Benelli suggests using a circular incision around the areola, removing excess breast tissue, leaving a cone of remaining breast tissue, and giving an aesthetically pleasing result. But, a plastic surgeon has to be well-versed in this technique in order to achieve a reasonable outcome. Sometimes the technique causes more scarring and asymmetrical nipple areolar complexes. The technique that Madeline Lejour presents is liposuction of the breast tissue. This is fine for fatty breasts with minimal ptosis, or drooping, and sagging skin. However, if you have a significant amount of ptosis, you may need to have skin resection and occasionally return for skin removal. Consulting with a plastic surgeon well-versed in these techniques will help you decide what technique would be most appropriate for your type of breasts.

Patients with droopy, or ptotic, breasts will be discussed in the next chapter about breast lifts.

Figure 13-3.
Breast Reduction

Recovery Time	Risk Factor	Pain Factor	Cost Factor
Initial: 10 days *Complete:* 3–4 weeks	Minimal if the patient is in good health. Not recommended for patients who smoke.	Most patients go home on oral medication the day after surgery	Most insurance companies foot the bill, but with HMOs tightening the reigns, most patients are now having to pay anywhere from $4,500–$8,700

CHAPTER 14

BREAST LIFTS

P totic, or droopy, breasts are a real concern for many women. Weight loss, a
severe diet program, pregnancy, and breast-feeding can all contribute to the
development of droopy breasts.

The most common patient is one who has had two children and breast-fed.
After pregnancy and breast-feeding, the top half, or superior aspect, of the breast
loses some of its fullness due to involution of breast tissue. Some patients are luck-
ier than others and actually develop fuller breasts after pregnancy, but this is rare.
Breast-feeding is extremely important for the baby, and women shouldn't avoid
this important part of the nurturing process just because it affects the appearance
of the breasts.

The most common operation performed is the mastopexy. It involves repositioning the nipple areolar complex to a location higher on the chest wall. The incisions are located around the nipple areolar complex.

This operation is usually done under general anesthesia or heavy IV sedation.
It can be done as an outpatient procedure in a hospital operating room or in a
physician's operating room, and it takes approximately three hours.

On occasion, some patients will lose quite a bit of fullness to their breasts, and

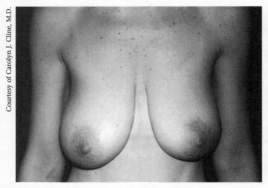
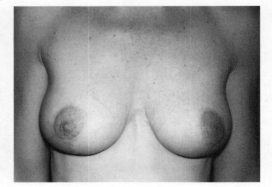

Courtesy of Carolyn J. Cline, M.D.

Figure 14-1. Before and after a breast lift mastopexy

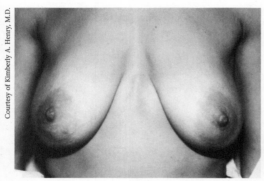
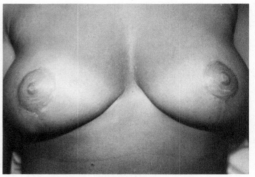

Courtesy of Kimberly A. Henry, M.D.

Figure 14-2. This thirty-two-year-old woman wanted fuller breasts that looked less droopy.

in addition to the lift, may require the placement of breast implants. (See Chapter 12 regarding breast implants.) In this case, the lift is performed in the usual way, and the implants are placed, most often, underneath the muscle. Some before-and-after pictures which depict the expected result postoperatively are shown in Figures 14-1 and 14-2.

Occasionally, other types of breast lifts will be recommended depending upon the degree of ptosis that is present. Your plastic surgeon will categorize your breasts with mild, moderate, or severe ptosis and make a decision about the type of operation (ultimately where the incisions will be) necessary to place your nipple areolar complex in the correct location.

Other techniques include the "crescent" mastopexy for mild ptosis and the circumareolar technique also for mild ptosis; the vertical scar technique for moderate ptosis; and the vertical technique (anchor incision) for the severe or major ptosis. (See Figures 14-3 to 14-6.)

Once a procedure is chosen, I describe it in detail to the patient. I let them know to expect red and noticeable incisions for up to a year and sometimes longer. If patients' expectations are realistic, they will be satisfied with their results.

After the operation, expect to be a little uncomfortable for a few days. Your doctor will usually recommend that you wear a bra or have a special dressing in place to provide the support you will need during your recovery. I sometimes ask my patients to wear a supportive Miracle bra or push-up bra that helps keep everything in place for twenty-four hours a day for at least four to six weeks. For the first week, you require pain medication. I routinely prescribe antibiotics as well. Your surgeon may have placed drains that need to be removed the second or third day.

If implants were placed, you will need to be careful to avoid impact-to-the-chest-type activities, as this may cause rupture of the implant.

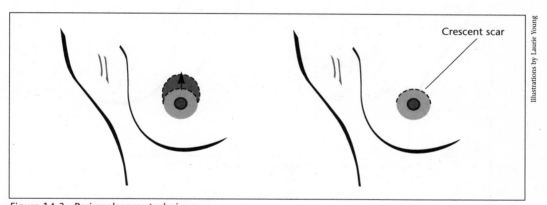

Figure 14-3. Periareolar scar technique

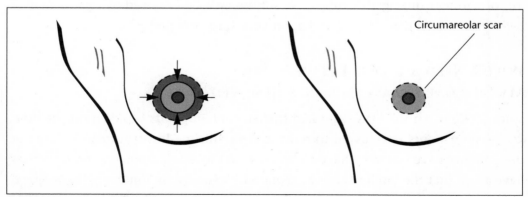

Figure 14-4. Circumareolar scar technique

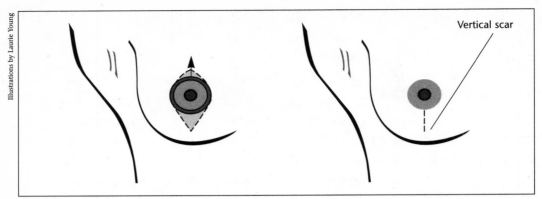

Figure 14-5. Vertical mastopexy scar technique

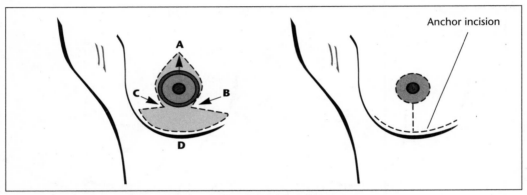

Figure 14-6. "Anchor" type incision, the most common type of mastopexy

Activity should be limited for four to six weeks postoperatively: no heavy lifting or aerobics during this time. The sutures will be removed at approximately seven to fourteen days, depending upon your surgeon's preference.

WILL I NEED A LIFT IF I HAVE MY SILICONE BREAST IMPLANTS REMOVED?

Since 1992, when the FDA requested that silicone implants be taken off the market, some patients have asked to remove their silicone breast implants. Some of the patients have opted to have them switched to saline implants, while others have asked that the implants not be replaced. On occasion, following the removal of the implant, it is necessary to do a mastopexy, or breast lift. The surgeon would use the same techniques as described above to help reposition the nipple areolar complex after removal of the breast implants.

WILL I EVER NEED A MASTOPEXY AGAIN IN THE FUTURE?

Yes, it is possible that you'll require another mastopexy or breast lift. Time moves on. Gravity will continue to take its toll on your body, and the aging process goes on. Sometimes a repeat mastopexy will be necessary as a "touch-up" procedure to improve the overall look and does not involve a full-length procedure.

In the next chapter, we will be discussing rhinoplasty, or nose surgery.

Figure 14-7.
Mastopexy—Breast Lift

Recovery Time	Risk Factor	Pain Factor	Cost Factor
Initial: 7 days *Complete:* 3–4 weeks	Minimal if the patient is in good health. Not recommended for patients who smoke.	Minimal to moderate. The addition of implants can increase discomfort.	$3,800–$4,800

CHAPTER 15

RHINOPLASTY, OR NOSE SURGERY

Reshaping the nose is one of the most rewarding operations requested in cosmetic surgery. Patients considering a rhinoplasty are usually unhappy with the shape or size of their nose, and may also desire a change in the tip, nasal bumps, size of the nostrils, or to correct a deformity or breathing problem.

While the Barbra Streisands and John Barrymores of this world have enjoyed promoting their famous profiles, the majority of people can easily find a multitude of sins in their noses.

When a patient comes to my office for a consultation about nose surgery, I suggest that he bring some pictures of noses along to the appointment. This way I can get some idea of the goals and expectations of the patient, and we can discuss the possible outcome of the surgery.

I perform nose surgery on patients of all ages, but the majority of them are in their late teens through their thirties. Many teenagers are unhappy about their appearance, feel awkward, and are constantly striving to find perfection. Since most growth spurts have usually occurred by the ages of seventeen or eighteen, I don't recommend performing this procedure before that time. However, it is also

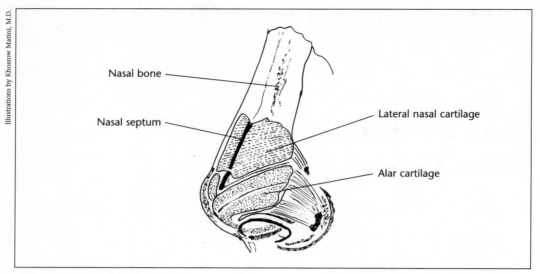

Illustrations by Khosrow Matini, M.D.

Figure 15-1. Nose anatomy

better for the patient emotionally to have this type of surgery at an earlier age since every year we live with our nose, it gets harder to think of changing our appearance. Therefore, if you are considering a change, the sooner in life, the better.

THE PROCEDURE

The procedure can be performed under local anesthesia with IV sedation or under general anesthesia. The operation takes anywhere from two to four hours depending upon the complexity of the procedure.

You should have had nothing to eat or drink after midnight the night before your operation. Plan to arrive at the hospital or surgery center about two hours prior to your procedure, since you may be asked to give blood for laboratory analysis or complete any extra paperwork. Before a rhinoplasty is performed, your physician will take "before" photos of your nose and to refer to during the surgery. This procedure is one of the most difficult to perform. It requires extra training and a lot of concentration and thought on the part of the surgeon. A thorough consultation with the patient, as well as these photos (and any the patient had brought to the consultation) will aid the surgeon in achieving the desired goals.

Once you are in the operating room, either the surgeon or anesthesiologist will administer sedation, depending upon the type of anesthesia you have requested. Surgeons will approach the rhinoplasty differently, depending upon their training and levels of expertise. For example, one surgeon may make only internal nasal incisions, incisions inside the nose, while another doctor might prefer the incisions outside the nose along the nasal tip, or columella (open-tip rhinoplasty). Each surgeon will have a technique that works well for him or her. Before any incision is made, the nose is anesthetized with local anesthesia (either lidocaine or marcaine with epinephrine). In addition, most surgeons use a combination of cocaine and/or epinephrine. This helps to shrink the mucous membranes as well as control bleeding. The surgeons then begin the operation using either the external or internal approach.

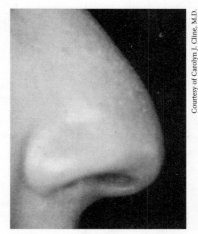

Courtesy of Carolyn J. Cline, M.D.

Figure 15-2. Before rhinoplasty

The nose is predominantly made of cartilage, and these are all exposed, as well as the small area of bony tissue at the top of the nose. The surgeon is then ready to sculpt these tissues. With the open-tip rhinoplasty approach, the surgeon has a greater opportunity to sculpt the nasal tip, making it more refined in appearance. Often, in nose surgeries, the patient can be left with an asymmetrical

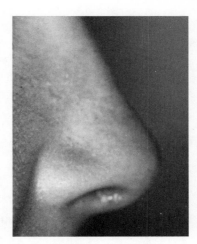

Figure 15-2. After rhinoplasty

or uneven tip. This is why the open-tip rhinoplasty is so pleasing because the surgeon is able to develop a symmetrical tip. Following the contouring of the nasal tip, the septum is sometimes straightened, depending upon whether or not you have an airway obstruction. Additionally, the top of the nose which often has bumps, can be revised either with a rasp or file or with a specific instrument called an osteotome used for contouring the nasal bony tissue.

Throughout the operation your surgeon will check the patient's profile on

Figure 15-3.
Rhinoplasty or Nose Job

Recovery Time	Risk Factor	Pain Factor	Cost Factor
Initial: One week with splint	Minimal if a patient is in excellent health	Feels like a bad cold	$3,000–$4,000
Complete: 6 months (final appearance)			

many occasions, the symmetry of the tip, and the improvement after each small change that is made. Rhinoplasty is a real art. Small changes consisting of 1 to 2 and up to 4 millimeters can make very large changes in the overall appearance of the nose. It is a delicate procedure and must be carefully performed.

After revising the cartilage, septum, and the top of the nose, the surgeon will often perform what we call osteotomies, where the actual bony tissue of the nose is broken and repositioned.

At the completion of the operation, the surgeon will recheck the size of the nostrils. Sometimes these openings have to be made smaller as in the case where the nostril base is quite wide.

Following this, small sutures are placed to close the incisions. Packing is then placed depending upon a surgeon's preference. Following this, a splint is usually placed on the nose and kept in place for about seven to ten days. The packing is usually kept in for twenty-four to forty-eight hours. A surgeon will prescribe some antibiotic medication as well as pain medication.

RECOVERY

When you go home, the surgeon will usually ask you to keep your head elevated for the next forty-eight to seventy-two hours, as this will help the swelling and help your overall well-being. You may feel a heaviness between your eyes and a little bit of a headache following the procedure. This is all normal, and it can improve with pain medication. Rarely do people experience significant discomfort, although, there are some patients that feel sore afterward.

You can expect to be black and blue around the eyes following rhinoplasty. This bruising will begin to dissipate within seven to ten days, and the splint is usually removed at this time. Cover-up makeup can be applied to improve your appearance.

Sometimes people combine other types of procedures with rhinoplasty, such as a chin augmentation or a malar (cheek) augmentation. This is an individual need and can be discussed with your surgeon prior to the procedure. In order to improve facial balance, most surgeons will recommend a chin implant if the chin is retro-positioned (positioned posteriorly).

After the splint is removed in approximately one week, your nose will continue to be swollen, but do not be discouraged. This is the worst that a new nose will look, but the patient is often disappointed at first glance. Be assured that in two to three weeks (longer in patients with open-tip rhinoplasties) you should be very pleased with the appearance of your new nose. It is very important that you do not accidentally bump your nose during this healing period. Small children may not mean to poke Mommy's or Daddy's new nose, but it can easily happen. I suggest staying more than an arm's length from kids and pets, and also recommend sleeping on your back.

If your surgeon has used nasal packing following the procedure, it will be removed after a few days. You may feel some stuffiness in your nose for several weeks, but resist the temptation to blow your nose.

About 17 percent of the time rhinoplasty revisions need to be performed. Sometimes small irregularities of the bony tissue or little bumps have to be refined, and this can usually be done under local anesthesia in an office setting.

After your surgery, there are several rules you should abide by. Besides avoiding bumping your nose, there are other guidelines you should observe. You can usually return to work or school a week or so after surgery, but avoid any strenuous activity such as swimming, high-impact aerobics, and sexual relations for at least three to four weeks. Avoid the sun on your nose, and don't rub too hard while washing your face. Eyeglasses or sunglasses should not be worn for six or seven weeks until the nose is completely healed, so I recommend contact lenses for this period. Remember, some swelling will be present for months, and the new nose may not have its final new look for up to a year.

In some cases, your insurance company may cover the cost of the nasal surgery. If your nose has been traumatized in an accident or if your breathing is dif-ficult due to a deviated septum, the insurance carrier will often take care of the sur-gical and facility fees. A consultation with your plastic surgeon and information and photos sent to the insurance company will clarify any coverage for the patient.

In the next chapter, we will discuss one of the most common plastic surgery procedures performed on both men and women today, liposuction.

CHAPTER 16

LIPOSUCTION

Liposuction is one of the newest and now the most popular form of cosmetic surgery. This procedure, also called suction-assisted lipectomy, uses a special suctioning device that permanently removes excess fat cells which have become localized in specific areas such as the thighs, buttocks, knees, calves, abdomen, and waist. Liposuction is most effective on areas where diet and exercise don't seem to work.

Liposuction is a technique that was first started in France approximately fifteen to twenty years ago. Since its initial development, it has evolved to subsets of liposuction to include liposculpture, the latest tumescent technique, and a very new technique currently under investigation and possibly available by the time of the publication of this book, called ultrasonic liposuction. Currently, liposuction is the main plastic-cosmetic surgery operation being performed today. This is not surprising, considering the amount of positive feedback I get from my patients. Some of my patients get such a boost from having the liposuction that they go on to lose more weight on their own.

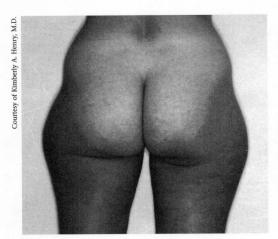

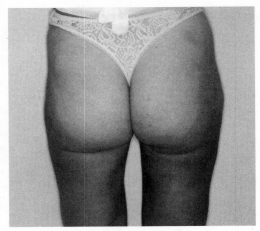

Figure 16-1. The patient at a size 14 before liposuction.

Figure 16-1. Now down to a size 6.

WHO IS A GOOD CANDIDATE FOR LIPOSUCTION?

The ideal patient is in good physical shape, has good skin tone, is not overweight, and has distinct localized pockets of fat that have been resistant to dieting and exercise in the past. Liposuction can help people lose those extra fifteen to twenty pounds that they just can't lose. While age itself does not affect the success of the procedure, the best results are found in patients under the age of forty, since their skin is more elastic; but liposuction can also be performed on older patients with good results.

I must caution that liposuction is not a cure for obesity nor is it a way to remove the dimpled skin commonly referred to as cellulite. There are some "superficial liposuction experts," though, who feel that cellulite and the dimpling associated with it can be improved with this procedure.

Liposuction can be performed on an outpatient basis under local or general anesthesia. The doctor makes incisions that are no more than one centimeter in length and placed in inconspicuous areas, so there is minimal scarring. With newer techniques, plastic surgeons are able to remove more tissue than ever before and with less bruising and swelling. Previously, they were limited to removing between 1,500 and 2,000 ccs. Now, they can remove 4,000 to 5,000 ccs without a blood transfusion on an outpatient basis, and often, patients can return to work and normal activity much sooner.

The recovery period generally lasts two to three weeks, but because of some residual swelling, the final result may not be visible for up to three to six months.

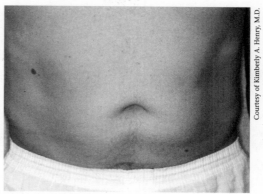

Figure 16-2. Before liposuction of the abdomen

After liposuction, you will be required to wear a restrictive outer garment resembling a tight girdle over the area where the surgery was performed. These garments help reduce swelling, compressing the skin as it goes through many changes. It is very important during this stage for the skin tissue to be supported and sculpted for the proper reshaping to occur. They are changed at the follow-up visits and at home.

In cosmetic surgery, as in every form of surgery, complications may sometimes arise. Complications are extremely rare, and the chances of developing a minor complication are about one in one hundred. Before surgery, your doctor will review your

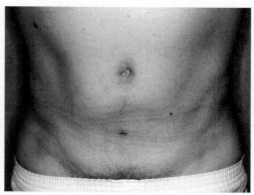

Figure 16-2. After liposuction of the abdomen

medical history, blood pressure, and any medications you are taking before deciding to proceed.

Remember, successful surgery also depends upon communicating your expectations and desires. It is important to discuss these things with your doctor so that realistic results can be achieved.

AREAS OF THE BODY HELPED BY LIPOSUCTION

Liposuction works best on the following areas: face, neck, breasts, arms, chest/breast (enlargement of the breast area in men), abdomen, hips, thighs, knees, and ankles.

A new technique presented in France by Madeline Lejour incorporates liposuction for the reduction of large breasts. It is routinely used in breast reductions by many plastic surgeons to help reduce fullness around the underarm and back area.

Dr. Patrick Maxwell, one of the country's leading plastic surgeons, is currently investigating the technique of ultrasonic liposuction for FDA approval. It is not yet available in the United States except through investigational studies; however, it is available in France and Italy. This technique uses two stages, beginning with an ultrasonic probe directed through the tissue that "breaks up" and emulsifies the fat. This is followed by a vacuuming of the liquefied fat. With this procedure, there appears to be much less trauma to the tissue than with other techniques. But, as with any new technique, the kinks still need to be worked out. Eventually, ultrasonic liposuction may replace current clinically-proven procedures for liposuction.

In the next chapter, we will be learning about lasers, the new space-age technology for plastic surgery.

Figure 16-3.
Liposuction

Recovery Time	Risk Factor	Pain Factor	Cost Factor
1–2 sites: 2–3 days *3 or more sites:* 7–10 days	Minimal in healthy patients. Must be performed by an appropriately-trained surgeon.	Minimal to moderate	$1,000–$2,000/ site. Most surgeons will discount for multiple sites. *Garments:* $50–$75/piece

CHAPTER 17

The Lasers

The laser is a space-age technology that has finally made its way to the plastic surgeon. Public interest in the Ultra Pulse CO_2 laser by Coherent Laser Corporation has taken off like wildfire. It was initially presented at a March 1995 conference at the Aesthetic Society of Plastic and Reconstructive Surgeons (ASPRF) in San Francisco. At that time, very few people were using lasers. Since then, however, more and more plastic surgeons, dermatologists, and general surgeons have begun to use Ultra Pulse CO_2. Its main benefit is to obliterate the fine wrinkling around the lips as well as the fine wrinkling around the eyes. This technique creates an energetic disruption of the orientation of collagen skin cells causing the collagen bundles to shrink and thus eliminating the wrinkles. No other technique in plastic surgery is able to achieve such wonderful results.

What Can Lasers Treat?

Lasers can treat the following:

- fine wrinkles around the mouth and around the eyes and cheeks
- tattoos

- spider veins around the legs, face, nose, cheeks
- some stretch marks on the legs
- age spots
- birthmarks

Laser works the best around the eyes and around the mouth. The "lipstick bleed" is, for the most part, eliminated with the laser. Fine wrinkling and "crepe" paper skin around and below the eyes can also be eliminated with the Ultra Pulse CO_2 laser rather nicely.

There are different types of lasers, and each one has specific treatment capabilities. Some lasers treat age spots, while others are better at treating birthmarks. The Ultra Pulse CO_2 laser is the main laser used to treat wrinkles. The latest laser sclero-laser treats spider veins of the legs and was recently introduced in August 1996.

When considering laser surgery, make sure you consult with a board certified plastic surgeon or a board certified dermatologist who has knowledge of the lasers and how they work.

My practice often conducts evening or weekend plastic surgery seminars for our patients that allows them to see how a laser works firsthand. We call it our "tomato and eggplant" show. With the help of our laser technician, we actually instruct laypeople on the use of the laser and, in a very controlled setting, allow them to use it on vegetables. It is very easy to use. The laser attachment is like a small pencil.

GETTING READY FOR THE LASER

Ultra Pulse CO_2 Laser: "The Wrinkle Laser"

Most surgeons who do laser surgery recommend that patients "prepare" their skin in advance with either Retin-A or an alphahydroxy acid product at least four to six weeks ahead of time. I ask most of my patients regularly use a glycolic acid or lactic acid so that they do not need to wait the extra four weeks prior to pursuing their laser treatment. Again, each surgeon has specific recommendations regarding this, so consult with him or her.

THE DAY OF LASER

Your doctor will ask you to arrive wearing no make-up for the laser treatment. Depending upon how extensive the area to be lasered will determine whether your physician will recommend IV sedation or a straight local procedure. (Intravenous sedation places you in a "twilight zone" where you essentially do not remember the procedure at all.)

If my patients undergo laser of a small area (eyes or mouth only), I perform the procedure under local anesthesia only. If we are doing a full-face laser for acne scarring or following a face-lift to improve the wrinkling not eliminated with the face-lift, I generally use IV sedation. Some physicians may use general anesthesia.

Following the laser treatment, we apply neosporin or bacitracin ointment. Some surgeons use special dressings that are supposed to stay on for about a week after laser, but most of the time, they fall off after the first or second day. Sometimes we switch the neosporin or bacitracin with straight petroleum jelly or Vaseline for those patients with a sensitivity to the antibiotic ointments.

For those patients with a previous history of oral herpes, it is important to cover them with Zovirax, an antiviral medication that helps prevent an active herpes infection before and following laser treatment.

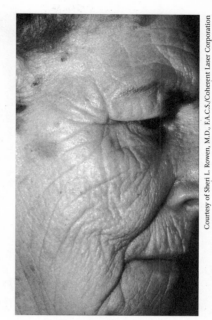

Courtesy of Sheri L. Rowen, M.D., F.A.C.S./Coherent Laser Corporation

Figure 17-1. Notice the severe wrinkling of the eye, cheek, and lip areas.

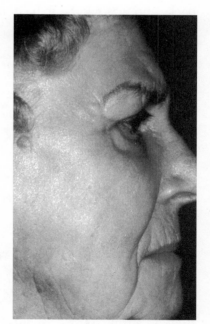

Figure 17-1. Laser resurfacing using Ultra Pulse CO_2 laser

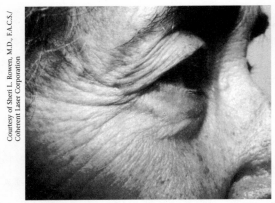
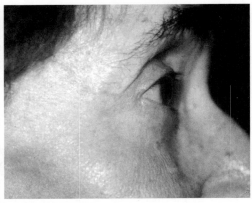

Figure 17-2. Laser resurfacing in conjunction with eyelid and facial surgery.

THE FIRST FEW DAYS AFTER SURGERY

Expect to feel a bit tired and worn out after laser. You'll feel like you have gotten the worst sunburn in the world. Your skin will feel tight, wet, and like it is on fire. We prescribe medication to help with the discomfort following the procedure. Ice packs and washcloths soaked in ice water are very comforting to the skin.

As someone who's had this procedure done, I'd say the first three to five days are the most difficult—you can't imagine that your skin will ever look good again, but, eventually it does. The wrinkles disappear, and you quickly forget those first early days and wish you had done it sooner.

After the fifth or sixth day, expect your skin to start peeling, and underneath, expect to find brand new pink skin that glistens and is as smooth as glass.

Your skin will remain red for anywhere from several weeks to several months, but this will slowly disappear. Most of my patients wear a cover-up make-up to help hide the redness postoperatively.

WHO'S A GOOD CANDIDATE?

Some patients are better candidates for laser resurfacing than others. Patients with dark skin or olive complexion should have a test patch with the laser before considering a full laser treatment. Patients with lighter skin tend to do quite well with laser treatment.

RISKS

As with any plastic surgery operation, one may encounter complications but there are very few related to laser. Complications following CO_2 laser may include pain and discomfort, swelling, change in skin color, scarring, infection, and recurrence of lesions. The quality of the skin following laser is variable and usually related to a person's genetic makeup. The treated area may heal either lighter or darker in color, but such pigmentation is usually temporary, though occasionally permanent. Solaquin Forte® cream after laser surgery helps lighten any darkened areas that many occur from sun exposure.

Unsightly scarring is rare, but some scars may be more visible than others. To reduce scarring, follow all postoperative instructions carefully, and notify the surgeon of any problems. Bleeding is also very rare; in fact, some laser surgeons treat patients who are taking aspirin and coumadin. But generally, patients on blood thinners are postponed until they can be off the medication.

Following the laser, the patients will have a severe sunburn for at least a week. Some patients choose to stay home during this seven-day period and relax, apply cool ice packs, and take medication for the discomfort. Most of the time, people are uncomfortable about going out because of the way their face looks, but this improves over time. It may take up to ten to twelve weeks for the redness to improve, so we provide our patients with cover-up make-up and professional instruction on its use.

Figure 17-3.
Ultra Pulse CO_2 Laser Resurfacing

Recovery Time	Risk Factor	Pain Factor	Cost Factor
7–8 days Redness can persist for several weeks, up to 5 months for some patients, but eventually disappears	Minimal if a patient is in excellent health. Patients must limit exposure to the sun. Winter, fall, and early spring are the best times to schedule laser resurfacing.	Moderate	$1,500–$6,000 plus the cost of anesthesia

TATTOOS: "THE BATTLESHIP HAS GOT TO GO!"

Tattoos are created when pigment is deposited in the dermis (the lower surface) of the skin. Some tattoos are professionally done, and others are done by amateurs. Tattoos sometimes have a stigma attached to them, and people will seek the services of a plastic surgeon to get rid of them.

Just a few years ago, we would have removed it by excising and creating a large scar. Now, with the invention of the new ND-yag laser, we can turn the laser "on," the energy light goes down into the tattoo and vaporizes the tattoo pigment. Some of the permanent cosmetic tattoo artists use our services to eliminate eyebrows and lip line permanent tattoos, while other tattoos need a second type of laser depending on the color of the tattoos. Occasionally, it takes more than one sitting to remove a tattoo. Check with your physician regarding fees for this.

The next chapter on dermabrasion discusses treatment for scarring, wrinkle lines, and tattoos.

Figure 17-4.
Tatoo Removal

Recovery Time	Risk Factor	Pain Factor	Cost Factor
Patients can return to work the same day	Minimal	Minimal—Local anesthetic is used	$300–$2,000 depending upon size of the tattoo

CHAPTER 18

DERMABRASION

Dermabrasion has been available since 1905 when a German dermatologist began using this technique for the treatment of post-acne scars.

Plastic surgeons currently use dermabrasion for the treatment of scarring related to acne, rhinophyma (the W.C. Fields nose deformity), chloasma (liver spots), acne rosacea, decorative tattoos, chicken pox scars, traumatic scars, multiple pigmented birthmarks, keloids, skin growths, and sun-damaged skin. It can help with the vertical lines of the upper lip, as well.

With the advent of the laser, we now have safer and more reliable techniques for removing tattoos, fine wrinkles around the lips, and scarring. However, dermabrasion is still performed and in some surgeon's hands works just as well.

THE ACTUAL PROCEDURE

Every surgeon has a specific way of performing dermabrasion. Some surgeons administer IV sedation prior to the procedure when they are doing a full face dermabrasion. Others will use straight local anesthesia if the area involved is limited to, say, a scar on the cheek.

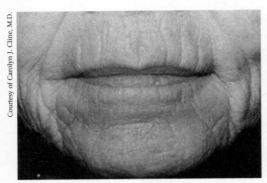 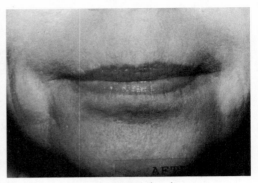

Figure 18-1. Dermabrasion for treatment of lines around the chin and mouth. Notice the close to complete elimination of the lines.

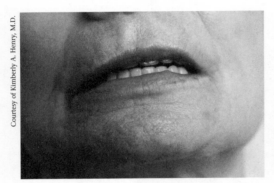 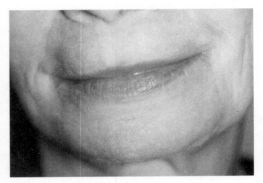

Figure 18-2. Chemical peel, dermabrasion, or laser can achieve the results above.

The skin is cleansed and prepared carefully. Some surgeons will actually freeze the skin with ice packs and then perform the dermabrasion. Some will apply 1 percent gentian violet solution to the face. Following this, the surgeon moves a rotating dermabrasion machine that is similar to a pencil with a small cone of metal sandpaper at the end of it around the areas of the face or skin that are involved with irregularities.

After the dermabrasion, expect your face to feel raw and irritated, similar to a skinned knee. Your skin will weep and drain serous yellow clear fluid, which is normal and expected. The first four to five days are the worst, and plan to "camp out" at home during the first week following your dermabrasion. Early on, your skin will be pink, red, and sunburned looking. Skin is brand new so wear heavy-duty sunblock and stay out of the sun. The new result, smoother skin, should be evident soon after your dermabrasion.

Occasionally, it will take up to eighteen days following a dermabrasion for full healing. A crust will automatically form during the early healing process, and this will need to be continuously removed with moist wet packs. If this is not done, the patient may develop a bacterial infection underneath the crust, which may lead to more severe scarring and worsening of their overall result.

RISKS AND BENEFITS

Sometimes, hyperpigmentation can occur postoperatively if a patient has been exposed to the sun for any length of time. In patients with active acne, dermabrasion needs to be postponed until the acne is quiet. Otherwise, a patient can develop a significant infection. Patients with a history of keloid formation are at risk of developing severe scarring following the procedure, as well.

Some evidence suggests that patients on Accutane may develop unusual scarring following laser or dermabrasion. Therefore, I do not recommend the use of Accutane for a long period of time prior to laser or dermabrasion.

The goal for any patient should be "any improvement at all." Most patients should expect at least a 50 percent improvement, and it may go as high as 85 percent. But knowing, again, that plastic surgery is improvement not perfection will help you accept your improved result following dermabrasion.

CHAPTER 19

COLLAGEN AND OTHER INJECTABLES

The Collagen Corporation based in Palo Alto, California, has been the main supplier of synthetic injectable collagen for years. The newer products, Zyplast and Zyderm, have been used to help increase the size of small lips, eliminate the line around the borders of the lips of smokers, eliminate the wrinkles of those with heavy sun exposure, eliminate acne scarring and acne pits, and treat the lines around the eyes and between the eyebrows.

Collagen is a nice way to begin the "appearance medicine" journey. Many people are sometimes frightened by the idea of plastic surgery. It's scary, it's real surgery. With collagen, those who are frightened can experience the joy following elimination of bothersome wrinkles and improvement of long-time acne scars.

Before you begin collagen therapy, it's necessary to have a skin test prior to the full correction of a line or acne scar. This test consists of injecting a small amount of collagen underneath the skin of your arm and watching for a period of three weeks to see if you have a reaction to the collagen. Most people who are allergic to beef will have some type of reaction to the collagen since collagen is made from bovine collagen. A red bump at the site or a rash is a positive reaction against the

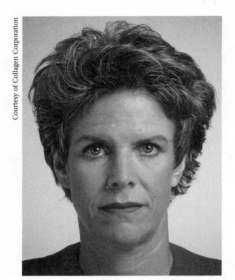

Figure 19-1. Before collagen injections

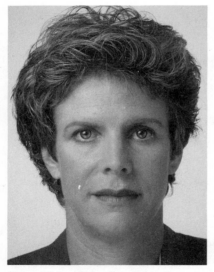

Figure 19-1. After collagen injections

collagen. Your surgeon or dermatologist needs to be notified right away of any type of reaction or problem.

If your skin test is negative, your surgeon or doctor can proceed with the collagen injection. Usually 1 to 3 ccs of collagen is injected. Each syringe costs anywhere from $350 to $500 per cc injected.

Following the injection, you will be swollen and a bit bruised. When I inject lips to augment them, I usually use the bulkier, more robust collagen zyplast. This is crosslinked (strands of collagen hooked together) and provides, along with heavier, bulkier collagen, to fill the line or depression. It will also last longer, anywhere from four to six months. Sometimes, after several injections, a patient will develop so much scar tissue in the area that scar buildup will further improve the look in addition to the collagen.

There has been some suggestion that patients may develop autoimmune disease following the use of collagen. This is currently under investigation. If you are concerned about this, refer to the collagen pamphlet which is provided before the procedure and thoroughly discuss this with your surgeon.

OTHER INJECTABLES

Other injectables include autologous fat (a patient's own fat), silicone (uncommon and illegal in the United States), and Fibril products. Sidney Coleman, M.D., and some doctors in Sweden have developed beautiful techniques using a patient's own fat. Fat is removed from another part of the body and injected into areas of the face to help improve the effects of aging. As we age, our body and our face starts to lose fat in specific areas, specifically around the eyes and the cheek areas, causing the face to droop and sag. The injection of a person's own fat in specific areas of the face helps rejuvenate the face.

Before 1992, silicone gel injections were used exclusively to augment the face. At this point, they are currently banned by the FDA due to frequent complications. The silicone was known to migrate to different parts of the face causing it to look very lumpy.

Every type of injectable may cause infection. Every type of injectable may reabsorb, requiring repeat injection in the future. For most people, this technique is worth it.

In the next chapter, we will discuss the latest in lip augmentation.

Figure 19-2.
Injectables

Recovery Time	Risk Factor	Pain Factor	Cost Factor
24–48 hours	Minimal but may need to be replaced	Minimal	*Collagen:* $350–$500/syringe *Fat injections:* $1,500–$2,000–$4,000 *Fibril products:* $500/syringe

CHAPTER 20

Lip Augmentation and Reduction

S ince the latter part of the last decade, larger, pouty lips have been fashionable. Movie stars like Kim Basinger and Barbara Hershey fit the bill just perfectly. But what if you missed out on the genes that provided such enhancement—what can a plastic surgeon do to improve upon thin lips?

Collagen

Perhaps the most common and easiest of all the procedures to enhance the lips is collagen injections. Most plastic surgeons will use Zyplast, which is a "bulkier" collagen that tends to last longer once injected. All patients will require a skin test beforehand to determine if they will have an allergic reaction to the collagen. (See Chapter 19.)

The overall procedure of injecting the lips with collagen takes at most twenty to thirty minutes and is done under local anesthesia. Expect to be swollen for the first sixteen to twenty-four hours. Some of the swelling will then subside and you will have new enhanced beautiful lips. Occasionally, there is a little bruising from the injections. The fullness of your lips will last anywhere from three to six

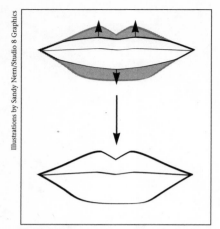

Figure 20-1. Lip lift. An incision is made around the outline of the lip, the gray area is removed, and the lip tissue is stretched and stutures into place

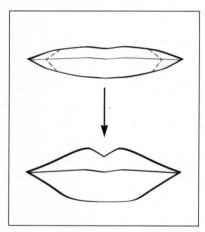

Figure 20-2. Alloderm. Small incisions are made on both the upper and lower lips and Alloderm is threaded across the lips.

months. Your body will naturally degrade the collagen over time. Multiple injections of collagen may cause scar tissue to form which will make the lips seem even fuller. Instead of being full with collagen, they are full with scar tissue. However, it's unclear if this occurs in all patients.

GORTEX

The parka material used for our winter coats has now become useful in the operating room. Gortex can be used for the treatment of hernia repairs and to repair blood vessels. Cosmetic surgeons can also use it to enhance noses, chins, cheeks, and lips. One prominent Los Angeles surgeon threads three to four strands of Gortex suture under the skin very easily to create bulk in the area of the lips. The whole procedure takes about thirty minutes, and there are minimal risks involved. Occasionally, the material can become infected and will need to be removed.

FAT INJECTIONS

Dr. Sydney Coleman, a well-known New York plastic surgeon has probably the most experience using fat injections to augment the face. (See Chapter 19.) It is very easy to remove unwanted fat from another area of your body (the best location is your inner thigh region) and reinject it to re-create fullness in the lips. Again, there is always the possibility of fat reabsorption (called resorption, where the fat is *re*-absorbed by the body) where the body slowly dissolves the fat leaving none.

DERMAL FAT GRAFTS

Other techniques include removing tissue (fatty tissue and dermal skin tissue) and surgically placing it under the skin of the lips to create fullness. This procedure takes approximately one hour and can be done under local or general anesthesia.

LIP LIFT

The most involved procedure for lip augmentation is a lip lift. In this procedure, a "new lip" border is outlined, and skin from the actual red border of the lip is moved to the "new lip" location (see Figure 20-1). Sutures are left in place for seven days. Again, the recovery is relatively easy.

ALLODERM

The latest in lip augmentation over the past eighteen months, plastic surgeons have been using Alloderm, a new type of implant material, for augmentation to help improve depressed scars and to plump up lips. The implant material is developed from human tissue and is thought to eliminate former rejection problems seen with other materials, allowing it to last longer, if not forever. The Alloderm is delivered in a "freeze-dried" form to the surgeon's office. It is prepared and then is ready to be implanted. Small incisions are placed in the corners of the mouth and the Alloderm is threaded through the lip. (see Figure 20-2). The openings are sutured closed. Sutures remain in place for seven days. Patients can expect to be very swollen for the first week, but this gradually improves. According to some surgeons there may be less trauma to the tissue with Alloderm than with collagen. However, the placement of Alloderm is more involved and more expensive than collagen injectables.

MAKING LIPS SMALLER: IS IT POSSIBLE?

Some patients are bothered by the size of their large lips. A few operations can help thin out the lips and make them smaller. Under local anesthesia or IV sedation, a wedge resection of excessive lip tissue is performed (the reversal of a lip lift). The patient has sutures in place for approximately one week. Lips will remain swollen for several weeks, but a patient will notice an overall improved appearance of the size and shape within the first week.

Figure 20-3.
Lip Augmentation and Reduction

Recovery Time	Risk Factor	Pain Factor	Cost Factor
Lip Lift or Reduction: 7 days with sutures in lip	Minimal if patient is in excellent health	Minimal	$2,500–$3,500
Collagen: 24 hours *Fat Injection:* 72 hours *Gortex:* 24 hours *Alloderm:* 4 days	Minimal risk of infection, somewhat higher with Gortex	Minimal	*Collagen:* $350 *Fat injection:* $600–$1,500 *Gortex:* $750 *Alloderm:* $2,500

CHAPTER 21

Abdominoplasty, or Tummy Tuck

The abdominoplasty is a surgical procedure to remove excess skin and fat from the abdomen and to tighten the muscles of the abdominal wall. Good candidates for a tummy tuck are patients who have developed laxity in the skin and muscles of the abdomen and stomach areas. After several pregnancies, a Cesarean section, or large weight loss, many women are ready to make a call to their plastic surgeon. More and more men are also opting for this procedure, and it is becoming increasingly popular. This procedure does produce a permanent, noticeable scar; however, it is one that is easily hidden by clothing. The scar is placed in a low crease in the abdomen or stomach skin.

Most people who seek abdominoplasty are either somewhat overweight or have a lot of skin redundancy following either a large weight loss or a pregnancy. In the case of pregnancy, the muscles of the abdominal wall separate and and then stretch considerably as the child grows inside the womb. Following the birth of the baby, this tissue involutes but does not return to its original laxity and tautness. Women who have multiple births have an even harder time regaining the original laxity and tautness of the abdominal wall. Often, these mothers are potential candidates for a tummy tuck. Many men who have gained a considerable amount of weight and then lost most of it want to tighten up their abdomens and remove the excess skin and fat. We must stress that women who plan to have more children should put off having this procedure done until after any future family planning since the abdominal muscles that are tightened during surgery can separate again during another pregnancy. Also, the tightened muscles from an abdominoplasty can cause restrictive growth of the fetus.

When the patient meets with the surgeon for a consultation, the doctor will evaluate the amount of fat deposits in the abdominal area and will check the skin tone and basic health of the patient. There are several methods used for eliminating fat in this area of the body.

OPTIONS

1. *A mini-tummy tuck*
   This is done when most of the extra fat is below the navel, and this procedure can be performed on an outpatient basis.
2. *A complete abdominoplasty*
   This is usually necessary for people who have fatty deposits above the umbilicus, or belly button, as well as below the umbilicus in addition to excessive skin.

The abdominoplasty can also be used in conjunction with liposuction. In most cases, insurance companies do not cover the cost of this procedure, but you can always check with your insurance carrier to be certain. Some patients who have had previous abdominal wall surgeries and developed hernias in the location of the incisions may be able to get some of the procedure covered for repair of the umbilical or incisional hernia.

Newer techniques are currently being evaluated by some surgeons using the endoscopic approach. This is usually reserved for patients with minimal skin redundancies who may have some abdominal wall laxity that can be improved with the endoscope and by securing the muscles in place through small, tiny incisions in the abdominal wall, eliminating the need for a long incision.

There are a few things to remember when preparing for your surgery. Avoid getting sunburned, especially on the stomach area, and *do not smoke* as this impedes healing and can lead to separation of the sutures.

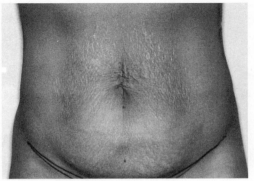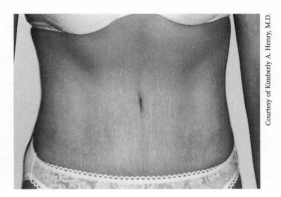

Figure 21-1. Before and after abdominoplasty

Courtesy of Kimberly A. Henry, M.D.

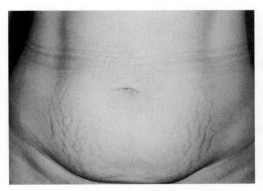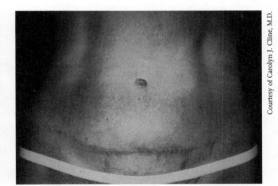

Figure 21-2. Before and after abdominoplasty

Courtesy of Carolyn J. Cline, M.D.

A full abdominoplasty procedure usually lasts from two to five hours, while a mini-tuck takes about one or two hours. An endoscopic abdominoplasty may take anywhere from three to four hours. Most physicians use a general anesthetic so that the patient is asleep throughout the procedure, while small tummy tucks or small liposuction procedures may only require local anesthetic with IV sedation. On some occasions, we can combine other procedures, such as a breast augmentation or breast reduction, with this one.

THE SURGERY

In most cases, the surgeon will begin by making the incision just above the pubic area extending out toward the hip area on both sides. Another incision is made

Illustrations by Khosrow Matini, M.D.

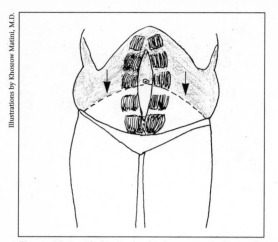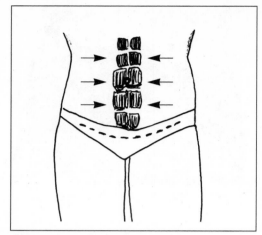

Figure 21-3. Abdominal muscles are pulled together, and excess skin and fat are removed.

around the belly button to remove it from the tissue and skin around it. (It will not be removed, just repositioned and is always attached to the abdominal wall.) The surgeon then lifts or separates the skin from the abdomen and elevates it up to the ribs so that the muscles in the abdomen are exposed. Next, the stomach muscles are tightened, pulled together to their original unstretched position, and held there by sutures. When this is accomplished, the skin flap is then brought back down, and excess skin and fat are removed. The navel is repositioned in a new spot and is sutured into place. At this point, the operation is completed, and the incisions are closed, dressings and/or bandages applied, and often drains are placed to drain excess fluid for the next twenty-four to forty-eight hours. The patient is usually kept in the hospital at least one night and may begin walking the following day. The patient is often crouched over for a period of ten to fourteen days while everything is healing.

Sutures on the outside of the body are generally removed in seven to eleven days, and the absorbable sutures under the skin will dissolve within four months. Some surgeons will have the patient wear an abdominal support garment following the procedure, as this will help protect the area and usually is comforting following abdominoplasty procedures. Some patients want to keep wearing it after the four-week period is over because they feel more comfortable with the added support.

Following this procedure, most people will notice an improvement in any back pain that they may have developed from the laxity of their abdominal wall.

I have seen this on numerous occasions with my patients. In fact, a very thorough scientific study revealed that reapproximating the muscles of the abdominal area significantly helps with discomfort in the lumbar spine region.

The incision stays red and noticeable for up to one to two years. Most patients are so ecstatic about the result and the improvement of the contour of their abdomen, they could care less about the noticability of the incision. Most one-piece bathing suits will hide this as will regular underwear.

A patient must not be involved with any heavy lifting or aerobic activity for four to six weeks following the procedure. Exercise may be done after the recovery period, but I would suggest avoiding rigorous aerobics, or jogging for up to eight to ten weeks. Sex may be resumed in four to six weeks.

It may take some time for you to feel like you aren't carrying a two-ton weight on your stomach area. People who are toned and in excellent physical shape prior to the surgery will have a much shorter recovery period. These patients often return to work in two weeks, while others may take longer to get back to normal activities.

In the next chapter, we will discuss arm, thigh, and buttock lifts.

Figure 21-4.
Abdominoplasty or Tummy Tuck

Recovery Time	Risk Factor	Pain Factor	Cost Factor
1–2 days in the hospital A mini-tummy tuck can be performed on an outpatient basis	Moderate— Not recommended for patients in poor health or for smokers	Moderate to severe	$4,000–$8,000 plus hospital and anesthesia fees

CHAPTER 22

Arm, Thigh, and Buttock Lifts

The quest for the "perfect" body no matter what persists in society. This is evident in the physical health industry where large numbers of health clubs and aerobic spas have been opened up across the country. Of all the plastic surgery procedures for men and women, liposuction happens to be the most common one performed here in the United States. We want to look as physically fit as possible. Well, this section is not about liposuction (but Chapter 16 should be read in conjunction with this one), instead, it is about the ultimate operation for body contouring. The operations discussed here are major operations and require an extensive recovery, but in the long run, they are very much worth the time and effort. Of all the body contouring procedures available to plastic surgeons, these probably give the most dramatic postoperative results.

Oftentimes when a person loses drastic amounts of weight, they will have excess skin remaining which will need to be treated by direct excision. The most common operations follow a drastic weight loss of from 60 to 150 pounds. The main operations are the abdominoplasty or tummy tuck, breast reduction, arm lift, thigh lift, and buttock lift. The main goal of each operation is to remove as much excessive skin as possible, reshape and recontour the area, and then close

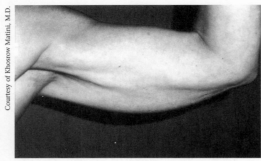 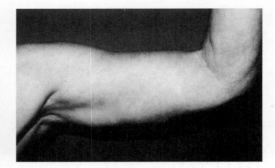

Figure 22-1. Before and after an arm lift

the incision in an inconspicuous location. The abdominoplasty and breast reductions were discussed previously. Please refer to Chapters 13 and 21. In this chapter, we will deal with arm lifts, buttock lifts, and thigh lifts.

ARM LIFT

I have numerous patients who complain about their droopy arms, especially when
summer arrives. During a consultation, they usually ask, while grabbing at the area
around their arm, "Now, isn't there something you can do about this?"

The procedure of an arm lift is relatively easy. The surgeon simply excises
whatever is hanging—excess skin and fat. These incisions are usually hidden
underneath in the inner arm area and extend from the elbow to the armpit.

The operation is done under IV sedation or general anesthesia. It takes anywhere from two to four hours to do the procedure.

Postoperatively, patients will be required to wear supportive Ace wraps for
about four weeks. Most patients are very happy with their results and care little
about the incisions, which may take up to a year to really mature. They are ecstatic about the overall new shape and size and how their clothes fit. They now feel
more comfortable in short-sleeved clothing.

The incision is made with some curvature and in the shape of a Z to decrease
the possibility of scar contracture and scar puckering. A curved Z-shaped incision
heals better in the healing process than does a straight-line incision.

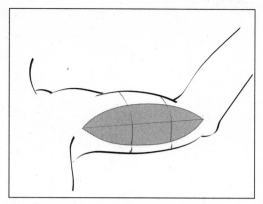

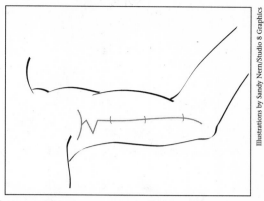

Illustrations by Sandy Nern/Studio 8 Graphics

Figure 22-2. Excess skin and fat is excised.

Figure 22-2. Curved and Z-shaped incision

Figure 22-3.
Arm Lift

Recovery Time	Risk Factor	Pain Factor	Cost Factor
Initial: 10 days *Complete:* 4 weeks	Minimal if a patient is in excellent health	Minimal discomfort	$3,500–$4,500 plus hospital and anesthesia fees

THIGH LIFT

This happens to be one of the more frequently-asked-for operations in my community, perhaps because people are so health-and-fitness conscious in California.

The inner thighs are probably the most difficult areas to improve upon when it comes to body contour surgery. Liposuction of this area helps make an improvement, but nothing that is exactly perfect. Other areas of the body do better with liposuction. Inner thigh lifts help improve the contour of the inner thighs.

Again, the same principle applies. Excess skin and fat are excised. The operation is usually done under general anesthesia and takes four to five hours to do both legs. Postoperatively, a garment is placed over the surgical site to give it support for four to six weeks. Once again, most patients could care less about the incision; their thigh contour is improved.

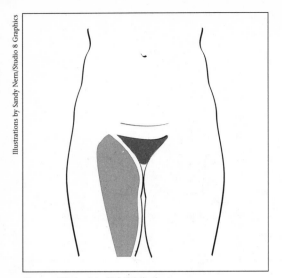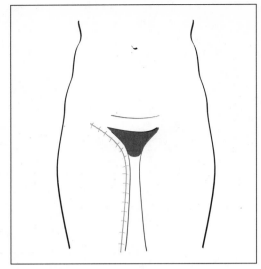

Figure 22-4. Medial thighplasty

BUTTOCK LIFT

Great candidates for a buttock lift are those with excess, droopy skin in the area just beneath the buttocks. Sometimes severe cellulite can be improved with this procedure as well.

It's relatively simple to excise excess skin and fat in this area. The incisions are hidden in the body crevices. The majority of these procedures are usually done at a hospital or surgery center under general anesthesia. The removed skin is discarded.

Postoperatively, the main obstacle to healing and recovery is not being able to sit. Patients are usually lying on their stomach the entire time during the first week. But gradually, as the incisions knit together, the patient can resume normal activity including sitting down.

Although complications are rare, the main ones are bleeding, infection, and scarring. Although wound disruption is uncommon, there may be some separation if you should sit on your incision or stretch it, and you may need a "touch-up" (scar revision) of the incision later.

Some people ask for liposuction when, in fact, they are, and mainly for age and genetic reasons, better candidates for thigh lifts or buttock lifts. If only liposuction is performed, the excessive skin would hang and look unattractive, and the patient would be back requesting a lift.

Figure 22-5.
Thigh Lift/Buttock Lift

Recovery Time	Risk Factor	Pain Factor	Cost Factor
Initial: 2 weeks *Complete:* 6 weeks	Minimal if a patient is in excellent health	Moderate	$4,000–$6,000 plus hospital and anesthesia fees

CHAPTER 23

CHIN AND
CHEEK IMPLANTS

Every time I see a Neanderthal man in the museum or in a textbook, I think of what I could do for him, specifically, his chin. Never mind his very prominent brow line. To reduce the size of a large chin takes a very thorough evaluation either by a plastic surgeon or an oral maxillofacial surgeon well versed in bimaxillary surgery (oral surgery of the cheek and chin region).

Facial balance is important when determining if someone has facial harmony. When you look at an attractive movie star, you are drawn to their facial harmony. The balance of their facial features makes them appear beautiful. Demi Moore, for example, or Sharon Stone, are excellent examples of facial balance. When a chin is small or set back, the proportions of the face in profile seem off balance. All of a sudden, the nose looks larger, the neck seems more obtuse, and the face does not seem to be in appropriate facial harmony or balance. The same is true when the chin is too large. A large chin on a man denotes strength and power—it is "masculine." However, the same chin on a woman would make her seem too masculine. With age, a chin can begin to droop and would be nicknamed a "witch's chin."

When I examine a patient for facial surgery, I am constantly interested in facial balance. I will check the profile from the nasal bridge, to the upper lip, and

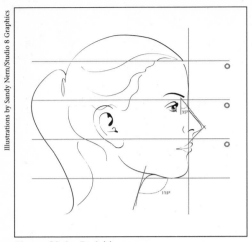

Figure 23-1. Facial harmony

to the most prominent part of the chin. The "line" I use should be close to a straight vertical. If it is skewed one way or the other, it will determine whether the chin seems too prominent or too retrusive (set back or small). It is almost a predictor of personality for some patients. Some men with smaller retrusive chins may be shier than men with larger chins; the same goes for women. After determining facial harmony, I make recommendations to patients regarding what would work best to improve their profile. Sometimes, it's placing a small chin implant, which is a relatively easy operation to perform with very little risk. Other times it's actually necessary to move the entire lower jaw forward, a more involved operation, but one in which the results are beautiful and dramatic.

WHAT CAN BE DONE WITH A SMALL CHIN?

If a chin is small, there are a few different ways to make it larger to improve the profile. The most common and probably the easiest for most surgeons, is to place a Silastic chin implant through a small incision inside the mouth or through an incision just under the chin in the small crease that most of us have. The procedure is relatively easy to perform, takes minimal time, and the recovery is relatively easy. After the operation, your doctor will instruct you to drink clear to full liquids for about ten days. There will be strict orders for minimal talking and laughing. Expect your lip to be swollen and uncomfortable for a period of time after the procedure if the incision is placed inside the mouth. It usually takes about five to six days to start feeling close to normal. Most patients will be placed on antibiotics for approximately ten days following the procedure. There are very few complications with this type of procedure; however, it is important that you keep following all instructions set forth by your plastic surgeon. Most surgeons recommend mouthwash irrigation every four to six hours. Infections are rare, but if they do occur,

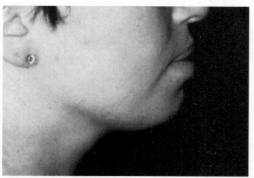 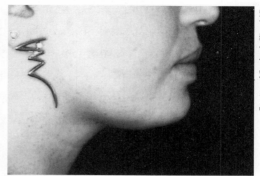

Courtesy of Carolyn J. Cline, M.D.

Figure 23-2. A chin implant adds definition and improves facial harmony.

patients are placed on antibiotics and usually improve over a short period of time.

The Silastic implant is made of firm, but soft silicone plastic. It is not made of silicone gel as with the silicone breast implants. At this point in time, there are no reports that chin implants cause any autoimmune diseases, and they are currently approved by the FDA to be used for plastic surgery patients. They are made from the same material that heart valves and hip replacements are made of. Other materials that are utilized as well are Porex and hydroxyapatite, just to name a few. Discuss this with your surgeon and find out which material he feels most comfortable with.

Some plastic surgeons use other types of tissue to augment or enlarge the chin. A well-known plastic surgeon in Los Angeles uses a person's own bony tissue and repositions the bone of the jaw forward, applying permanent fixating devices which help hold the new position in place. This operation is more involved, but it is necessary if a moderate amount of enlargement is necessary. The results following this procedure can be dramatic and well worth the extra recovery necessary.

WHAT ABOUT THE HUGE CHIN?

Jay Leno of the *Tonight Show* looks perfect with his large chin. It's part of his personality, and it suits him. However, if he got too close to a plastic surgeon, who knows what might happen?

A chin can denote strength and can be very desirable; however, if it seems out of proportion to the rest of the face, it may be necessary to "trim" some of the size of the jaw bone. This can be done through small incisions just inside the lower lip and just underneath the chin. Before any of this is done, however, your surgeon will spend time evaluating your photographs, X rays of your face, and your occlusion (bite) or how your teeth fit together.

First and foremost, we must evaluate how the teeth fit together. Some patients with really prominent chins have what we call a prognathic jaw line. In other words, their bottom teeth are in front of the upper teeth when the teeth come together. If this is the case, the jaw must be repositioned. Sometimes the plastic surgeon only needs to set back the lower jaw. Other times the upper jaw, called the maxilla, needs to be set forward because the lower jaw, called the mandible, is just fine, and it is the midface (the area of the cheek bones and upper lip) that needs improvement. Whatever it is, the chin needs a very thorough evaluation with X rays and the appropriate specialist.

If the dentition is fine and the teeth fit together well, then it becomes a relatively easy problem to correct. The bony tissue needs to be burred (literally) down to a size that is more cosmetically pleasing. This can be performed under general anesthesia or heavy IV sedation rather easily through an incision located just under the chin or inside the mouth.

WHAT ABOUT A NICE SQUARE JAW, LIKE CHRISTIE BRINKLEY'S?

The procedure of creating a square jaw line, similar to the many models you see on magazine covers, is one that has been around for about five or six years. The operation is for those that have a very long looking face and need some "facial width" in the lower aspect of their face.

The operation is performed under general anesthesia. Incisions are made inside the mouth along the lower aspect of the cheek. Small pockets are developed, and implants in the shape of an "L" are placed right along the side of the jaw bone.

Again, it's important to remain on liquids and soft foods for two to three weeks after the procedure. Most surgeons ask that any dental work be postponed for six months after placement of any facial implant. In addition, when dental work is performed, they recommend prophylactic antibiotics as well—preferably with a penicillin-type antibiotic—to be taken three to four hours before the dental work and approximately twenty-four hours following the dental work.

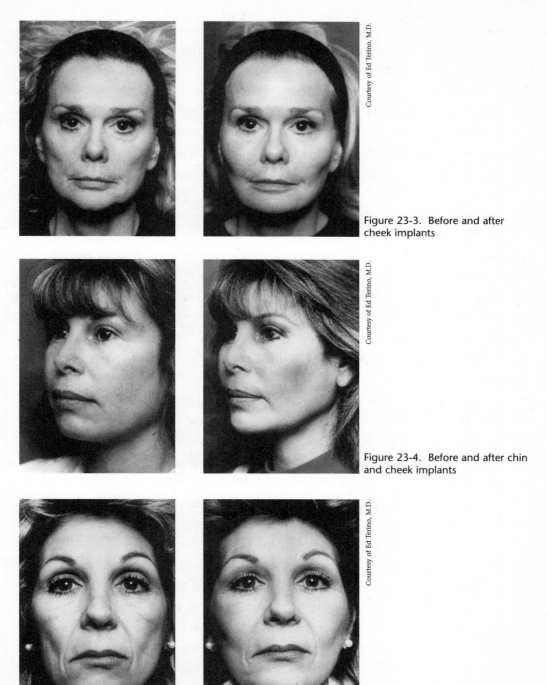

Courtesy of Ed Terino, M.D.

Figure 23-3. Before and after cheek implants

Courtesy of Ed Terino, M.D.

Figure 23-4. Before and after chin and cheek implants

Courtesy of Ed Terino, M.D.

Figure 23-5. Before and after chin and cheek implants

Facial Swelling: How Long Am I Going to Look Like a Chipmunk?

Major facial swelling improves in the first few weeks, but expect to have some persistent swelling for about two to three months. Expect your lip to be numb. It will feel like it doesn't belong to you, like when you are injected with Novocaine at the dentist, but this will all get better with time.

Expect to see a pleasant improvement in facial harmony following any one of these operations. A large majority of patients are extremely happy after these procedures.

CHEEK IMPLANTS

Prominent cheek bones like those of Cher, Faye Dunaway, and Janet Jackson are the current rave among plastic surgery patients these days. As a plastic surgeon, I can't help but notice faces all the time. When I'm at the grocery store, I study the *National Enquirer* like it was my homework assignment, and believe me, cheek implants have become one of the hottest and latest operations for those on the silver screen. It makes the face more youthful in appearance, less tired, less old, and gives them a new sense of vision.

As we age, we lose facial fat in the cheek area causing it to droop and hang down toward the mouth. The effect of this makes a person look tired, older, and sad. I have many patients in their mid to late thirties who come to see me with this concern, and in the past, we would have suggested a face-lift to lift the cheek and fatty tissue. With the development of cheek implants, we no longer have to recommend a face-lift as a first step. The cheek implant can be placed through an incision just inside the mouth. This creates a partial lift which helps create a more youthful, vibrant, healthy appearance to the face.

Eventually the patient will need a face-lift, and with some of the newer face-lifting techniques recommended by Steve Hoefflin, Jack Owsley, and Sam Hamra which specifically address elevating the cheek, we now know how important the architecture of the cheek fat is to the malar eminence (cheek prominence). Ed Terino, a well-known plastic surgeon in Los Angeles, has designed some of the facial implants currently on the market. He feels that implants provide much more dramatic and improved results when compared to some of the older techniques used.

The Operation

The surgery itself is usually done under general anesthesia or IV sedation. The surgeon will make small incisions inside the mouth near the cheek. Before the operation, they will mark your skin with the positioning of the implant.

Once a perfect pocket has been developed, the surgeon will place the appropriate-size implant in the area of the cheek. The incisions will be closed. Afterward, expect to stay on clear liquids and soft foods for three to four weeks. You will also be on antibiotics for at least a week. Following the operation, expect to be quite swollen for several days. It is very important to limit the amount of talking and laughing that you do. Most of my patients are instructed to limit the amount of tooth brushing using only a baby's toothbrush and to use a specific mouth rinse for several days at least three to four times a day. Facial swelling will set in, and expect to be swollen for three months. The initial swelling will diminish in about four weeks. You probably won't feel comfortable with your final appearance for another three months after the operation. You can't smile; your smile may be a little crooked initially; and it may not seem at all like you. However, with time, you can expect a full recovery.

Patients who have cheek implants placed are quite happy with the result. I can remember one patient who saw me weekly wondering when her chipmunk look would go away, and now she says it was well worth it. It is worthwhile, but the recovery can be prolonged.

Problems with Cheek Implants

It is extremely important that you remain on your antibiotics as prescribed by your surgeon. One of the most common complications following this procedure is infection. If, for any reason postoperatively, you develop drainage from the incision or redness and swelling around an implant, it needs to be evaluated by your surgeon. Dr. Ed Terino, who does the majority of cheek implant cases on the West Coast, states that he rarely has to remove the implant due to infection. Oftentimes if he suspects an implant is infected, he will tap the cheeks to see if he can express any fluid that may be sitting around the implants. This can easily be drawn off with a needle and syringe in the doctor's office.

Occasionally, the implants need to be repositioned. One may slide from its appropriate location. In this case it is very simple to remove the implant and reposition it in a more appropriate position. Discomfort from the cheek implants can occur, but it is rare and gradually improves with time.

In this chapter, we have reviewed the importance of facial balance and how to achieve it with augmentation using implants or reduction using bony tissue removal.

In the next chapter, we will be learning about men and plastic surgery and the two most common operations performed.

Figure 23-6.
Facial Implants and Surgery

Recovery Time	Risk Factor	Pain Factor	Cost Factor
Chin Implant: 5–10 days	Minimal if a patient is in excellent health	Mild/Moderate	$3,000–$4,000
Jaw Implants: 5–10 days	Minimal if a patient is in excellent health	Mild/Moderate	$5,000
Jaw Surgery: Up to 6 weeks	Moderate if a patient is in excellent health	Moderate	$5,000–$15,000
Cheek Implant: 7–10 days	Minimal if a patient is in excellent health	Moderate	$3,000–$4,000

MEN AND PLASTIC SURGERY:

Corporate America Is Waking Up

Over the past year the male population has made up approximately 10 percent of plastic surgery patients, and the number continues to increase steadily. It used to be hairdressers and actors who made up the majority of plastic surgery patients. Now, according to Dr. Daniel Baker, a plastic surgeon in New York, "Today I see investment bankers, lawyers, and business executives."

The most common procedures among men are, along with hair transplants (see Chapter 25) are eyelid surgery and liposuction. According to Dr. William Riley, a plastic surgeon in suburban Houston, "The eyes are it, as far as a businessman is concerned. His eyes are what he uses to meet his clients every day." One plastic surgeon has performed liposuction on pro football players to remove "love handles."

According to one part owner of a vending machine company in Houston, "Anyone who says he's not vain is a liar." He underwent surgery for his eyelids when someone said he had the body of a twenty-year-old, but the face of a ninety-year-old.

Figures 24-1 and 24-2 are a series of before-and-after pictures of men who have undergone plastic surgery. Pectoral implants, calf implants, and buttock implants are also being performed on men, but most of these types of operations are being

Courtesy of Khosrow Matini, M.D.

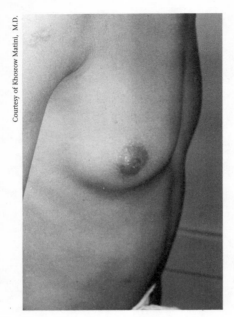

Figure 24-1. Gynecomastia, or excessive breast tissue, is common among men.

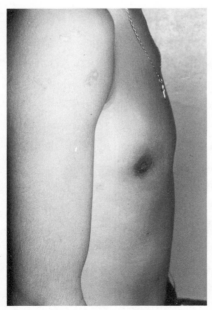

Figure 24-1. Liposuction can remove fatty tissue in the breast area.

done predominantly on the West Coast and in South America and only by a select few plastic surgeons. Other parts of the world do more aggressive, far-fetched-types of plastic surgery. Some of these operations include:

* reducing the size of the calves by removing muscles
* performing face-lifts on very young patients (in their twenties and early thirties)
* removing ribs from the rib cage to make the waist smaller
* using major craniofacial procedures to increase the projection of the cheek region or change the shape of the eyes

These atypical, aggressive procedures are more common in South America, Europe, Japan, and Thailand. Most plastic surgeons in the United States do not perform these operations.

WHY MEN HAVE EYELID SURGERY

The eyes are the pathway to the soul, or the focal point of the face and contribute substantially to a person's overall appearance. Most surgeons feel that more than any other cosmetic procedure the eyelid surgery helps a person look fresher and younger. It is by far the most popular cosmetic facial procedure performed today.

Bulging fat beneath the eyes, wrinkled skin, layers of skin under the eyelids and drooping eyebrows can give the entire face a

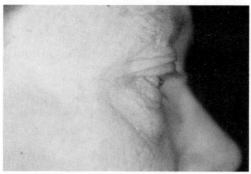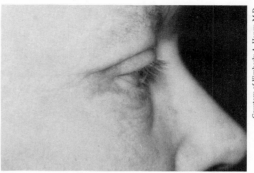

Courtesy of Kimberly A. Henry, M.D.

Figure 24-2. This man's vision was improved with eyelid surgery.

sad expression or a "mean" or "tired" look. Surgery can brighten a tired, or sad-looking face. In order to be competitive with a younger workforce, sell more commodities, close more houses, and "keep up" with the other guys, men will decide to have eyelid surgery.

MALE ENTERTAINERS

Beginning with Elvis Presley (who reportedly had a rhinoplasty according to *People* magazine), many male entertainers have considered and gone through with plastic surgery. The entertainment business is competitive. Most in the field opt for plastic surgery to keep up with the crowd. People think these actors and actresses have always looked this good. I often will buy *People* magazine and the *National Enquirer* just to keep track of what people have had done based on old photographs. I call it my "What has changed in this picture?" test.

PREPARE YOURSELF

With men becoming an increasing number of plastic surgery patients, we began to make some observations about them as a group.

First, the decision-making process is short. Once men decide on plastic surgery, their mind is made up. They don't have to talk about it or think about it like women tend to do. When they come in for a consultation for their eyes or liposuction and they have listened to the pros and cons, they make their decision, and move forward with their plans.

Second, they think that plastic surgery is like getting a haircut, no big deal . . .

until the day after surgery. I remember one gentleman in particular who underwent a face-lift, blepharoplasty, and abdominoplasty. The second day after his surgery, we helped him up to walk down the hallway at a hospital and his main comment was, "I didn't realize that I was going to feel wiped out." Therefore, prepare yourself. It's not a haircut, but it is worth it. Your surgeon will provide you with medication to help you with your discomfort, but it will take a few days or weeks before you feel like a million bucks. Just remember, you'll have to take it easy afterward.

If a wife, girlfriend, or relative cannot be with you initially, I recommend some hired help for a few days until you've gained your strength back. Expect to be swollen, and expect to be black and blue.

Third, plastic surgery can be as addictive for men as it is for women. They see the benefits. They, too, experience improved self-confidence. I've had several men who've returned interested in further plastic surgery because they were so happy with their first plastic surgery operation.

Fourth, men obviously do not make up the majority of plastic surgery patients. Initially, the idea of it all may seem quite uncomfortable to them, but when they see or talk to others who have gone through it, they feel more comfortable.

The next chapter discusses hair transplants for an overview regarding the latest procedures.

CHAPTER 25

Hair Transplants

By Miguel Delgado, M.D.

B aldness is universally uncomfortable for most men. Historically, as far back as 5000 B.C., man has been trying to develop a cure for baldness. Eventually, time and technology have provided man with a real solution. We now have a natural-looking hair transplant technique that has replaced the "hair tonics" of yesterday and the more recent "hair plug" telltale look of a "hair transplant."

Why We Go Bald

There are many reasons why a person may go bald: illness, poor nutrition, chemotherapy. Some patients develop alopecia (baldness) for no known reason. The most common reason men go bald is the male-pattern baldness gene. This requires a genetic inheritance from either the mother or father. The male-pattern baldness gene will be expressed if, and only if, there are normal levels of testosterone present in the bloodstream. Hair follicles around the sides and back of the head are not affected by this gene, so the hair can be transplanted from these locations and repositioned in the bald areas. The hair transplanted in the new location will grow

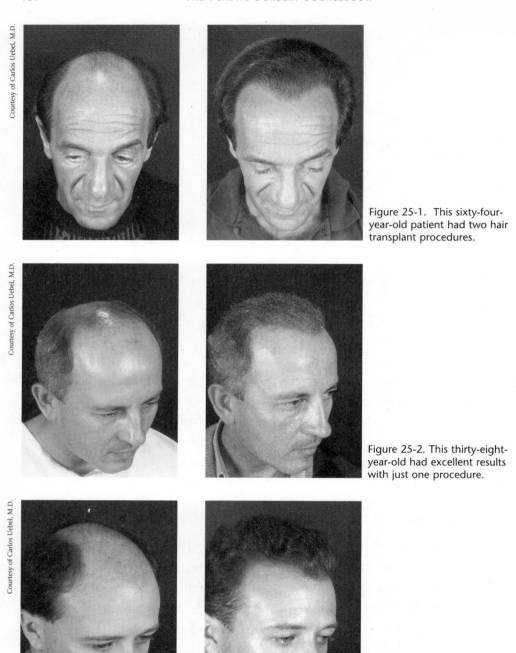

Courtesy of Carlos Uebel, M.D.

Figure 25-1. This sixty-four-year-old patient had two hair transplant procedures.

Figure 25-2. This thirty-eight-year-old had excellent results with just one procedure.

Figure 25-3. This twenty-eight-year-old patient had two micrograft procedures.

eliminating the baldness in these areas. If, however, one has generalized thinning all over the scalp, then one is not a good candidate for hair transplantation.

WHAT TYPES OF HAIR TRANSPLANTS ARE AVAILABLE TODAY?

Micrografts

Hair loss treatment is most commonly performed for men with acquired male-pattern baldness. In certain occasions, it is also available for females who have hair thinning in the anterior area due to various types of alopecia. But, men are the primary recipients of hair transplants today. In a specialized case of male-pattern baldness, one can change the posterior portion of the scalp and its normal hair-bearing state by transplanting varying amounts of hair from the anterior hairline back to the crown.

Micro and minigraft techniques are the most successful treatment modality for male-pattern baldness. This procedure minimizes scarring and provides the patient with instantaneous long-term results that won't vanish over time. Microsurgical hair grafts consist of one to five hairs and are taken from the back of the scalp and surgically placed into the bald area using a small incision. The remarkable small size of these grafts provide the patient with a natural appearance. Due to these technological advancements, microsurgical hair grafts alleviate the "corner row" or "doll's head" appearance that has long stigmatized hair replacement surgery.

Scalp Reduction

Another technique used in hair replacement surgery is the scalp reduction, a technique that reduces the bald area by direct excision and removal of scalp skin. This is usually accompanied with future micro and minigrafts.

Scalp Extension

The scalp extension is a flat rubberband-like device placed below the scalp to stretch the hair-bearing area. This is also used in conjunction with scalp reduction to accelerate the rate in which one can excise the bald scalp.

Tissue Expansion

In tissue expansion, we surgically place a balloon-like device underneath the part of the scalp that contains hair. The balloon is then expanded weekly. This stretches the hair-bearing scalp to two to three times its length and width. We can then almost excise the bald scalp area and relocate the "expanded" hair-bearing scalp into the area of baldness.

Scalp Rotation

The scalp rotation technique rotates the hair-bearing skin from the back and sides of the scalp to the front or anterior portion of the scalp.

The best technique for you is up to you and your surgeon.

ADVANTAGES AND DISADVANTAGES
OF EACH TECHNIQUE

One of the advantages of scalp-rotation is that when micro and minigrafts are placed, the hairs actually fall out once they're transplanted. They regrow after two or three months, and they never stop growing after that. However, with scalp rotation or other types of scalp flaps, the hair within the flaps do not go through a stage of hair loss. As one goes from micrografts and minigrafts, which are fairly simple office procedures, to scalp flaps and tissue expanders, these are more extensive procedures which entail more invasive surgery. The great disadvantage of tissue expansion is that one has to have large balloons underneath the scalp for approximately eight weeks.

TIME OFF WORK: WHEN CAN I GO
BACK TO MY JOB LOOKING REASONABLE?

The recuperation time depends upon the technique that is done. Typically after the micro and minigraft procedure, a head turban is placed for twenty-four hours. When this is removed, and the grafts are cleaned, the hair is combed, and neosporin is placed on the graft site. Over the course of the next week, the small scabs around the micrografts fall off, and vitamin E is usually applied to help wound healing. Once this is done, the micro and minigrafts appear as small pinkish dots which gradually fade within the scalp over a period of weeks. As stated earlier, the hairs extrude and fall out after about ten days, but this is followed by hair regrowth after about two to three months.

One should be able to go back to work once the turban is off. Wearing a hat is optimal until all scabs have been removed. The recuperation for scalp reduction and scalp extenders is similar. Once the procedure is performed, the sutures are typically removed in about ten days and replaced with a bandage. During that time, patients can wear a hat and can style their remaining hair over the operated site.

The tissue expansion procedure, which is performed less commonly today, has a longer recuperative period. This is a more invasive procedure usually performed under IV sedation or general anesthesia. Tissue expanders are placed near the back of the scalp, extending from ear to ear. Once the incision has healed, the expander is inflated over a period of approximately eight weeks. This requires weekly visits to the doctor's office for inflation. The difficulty begins when the tissue expanders become large enough whereby there is a noticeable difference in the size of the posterior scalp. The expanders are removed after eight weeks. The non-hair-bearing skin is excised, and the hair-bearing scalp tissue is advanced for coverage.

Depending upon the procedure performed, one can expect to look fairly normal early on. In general, once grafts are placed, the healing phase is short due to the size of the grafts, and cover up is extremely easy. A scalp rotation flap or tissue expansion, on the other hand, is a little more difficult.

HAIR TRANSPLANTS WITH BROW LIFTS AND FACE-LIFTS

Hair replacement surgery is also good for defects in the scalp that are due to either trauma or postoperative scarring. I sometimes see patients interested in improving the hair growth near a face-lift scar or a brow lift scar. Very often, the area of scarring has a fair amount of tension where a scar revision does not substantially improve this area, and hair grafts will certainly camouflage it extremely well over time. The minigrafts and the micrografts do require a fairly good blood supply.

CAN YOU MAKE EYEBROWS?

Hair transplant is also used to create eyebrows. This is a very well-known technique where one, two, or three fine hairs from the lower portion of the posterior scalp (the back of the head) are transplanted into the eyebrow area. The science today is so precise that patterns and shapes of eyebrows are predetermined as well as the direction of the hairs. Hair transplants are also being done on eyelashes.

How Expensive Are Hair Transplants?

The cost of micro and minigrafts depends upon where it's being done and who is doing it. Cost ranges anywhere between as low as $4.00 to $5.00 per graft over a certain amount of grafts to as high as $28 per graft. The scalp flaps are considerably more expensive due to the degree of invasiveness. A flap procedure, such as extended scalp flap, with all of the ancillary procedures, will cost anywhere between $5,000 and $10,000. A scalp reduction is typically in the range of $1,500 to $2,800. A scalp extension technique may add another $500 to $800 onto the scalp reduction cost.

The wide range of costs for all of the procedures is principally due to the degree of training acquired by the individual and the degree of personalized care. The procedures, in particular the mini and micrografts, are quite tedious, and splitting hairs into one, two, three, or four segments is quite time-consuming and needs to be done in a precise, meticulous fashion.

Rogaine: The Twentieth Century's "Snake Oil" Treatment for Baldness

One third of the patients using Rogaine or Minoxidil will have absolutely no response; another third may show an indistinguishable difference; and the last third may show some slight improvement. Overall, it will not "regrow" hair if one has some thinning or is in the early stages of hair loss. It may, however, slow down loss, and in some cases, it may increase the caliber of the hair. In a patient with a large degree of hair loss, it will do nothing more than grow peach fuzz-type hair over the hair-bearing scalp.

It is excellent for the very early hair-loss patients. It is also used by hair transplant surgeons after hair mini and micrografts to "fertilize" the regrowth of hair.

There are various Chinese vitamins that are used to basically increase the growth of hair, but none, however, is available for regrowth in the male-pattern baldness patient.

WHO SHOULD I TALK TO
ABOUT A HAIR TRANSPLANT?

Many physicians perform hair transplantations. Large hair clinics around the country have extremely extensive advertising and marketing campaigns that are city to city and who specialize in hair transplants. With many of these large clinics, the treatments are performed by various types of physicians who may be dermatologists, general surgeons, or even medical doctors. And the majority of the procedures will be performed by trained nursing staff.

The care and treatment by most plastic surgeons certified by the American Board of Plastic Surgery is generally more personalized. A board certified plastic surgeon has extensive surgical training and is adept at performing all of the male-pattern baldness techniques. You may or may not find a board certified plastic surgeon in one of these larger commercialized clinics. In addition, a plastic surgeon can also perform facial surgery to balance out the face as well as address concerns regarding baldness.

The most important thing when deciding on a hair-transplant surgeon, is to talk to his patients, get a comfortable feeling for him and his office, and determine what type of personalized care you will receive before surgery, during surgery, and after surgery.

Miguel Delgado, M.D., is a practicing plastic surgeon in San Francisco. His primary interest is male-pattern baldness and its treatment.

CHAPTER 26

Permanent Tattoo for Lips, Eyebrows, Eyeliner, and Battleships

Cosmetic tattoo salons are popping up all over my community in California. When I first started plastic surgery training in Oregon, I remember one of my first face-lift patients had tattooed eyeliner and lipliner. She was a rodeo rider and didn't want to take the extra time needed to get her makeup perfect. Well, that was about twelve years ago. Our society has gotten busier and busier; we have less time to put on our makeup.

At first, I thought women were rather brave to have makeup color permanently placed, but since my introduction to it five years ago, my feelings have changed. I have had my lips tattooed, and I am now considering having eyeliner placed, as well.

For some patients, the lip tattoo can decrease the evidence of lip bleed. Sometimes it creates more definition to the lip line that seems to disappear with age. Patients with lip scarring can actually be helped with colored lip tattoo. The tattooed pigment helps camouflage the scar and re-create a lip line that has been destroyed by injury. Patients with faint eyebrows, no eyebrows, or loss of part of an eyebrow, can benefit significantly from cosmetic tattoos.

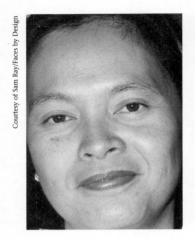
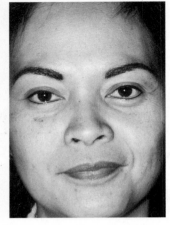

Figure 26-1. Eyebrow tattoos

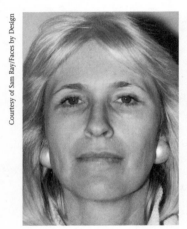
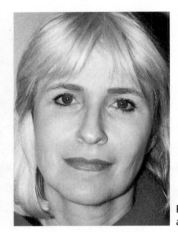

Figure 26-2. Eyebrow, eyeliner, and lip color tattoos

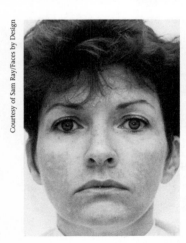
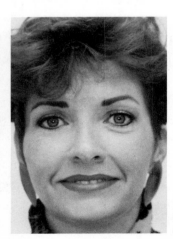

Figure 26-3. Eyebrow, eyeliner, and lip color tattoos

The Process

The procedure will either be done in a cosmetologist's office or in a plastic surgeon's office. Some plastic surgery nurses are trained to do the cosmetic tattoo as well. When you are deciding, ask to see pictures and talk to patients who have been through the process.

The anesthetic is usually topical, but occasionally, straight local anesthesia can be injected into the area. Some tattoo artists will have an agreement with a physician to inject with local anesthesia for those patients who can't tolerate the procedure under topical anesthetic.

Following the local, the area is then tattooed with specific pigment. There are many colors from which to choose for the lips, the brow, and the eyeliner. We also use the same pigments to tattoo nipple-areolar complexes following reconstruction for breast cancer.

Following the procedure, expect the area to be swollen for one to two days, Neosporin ointment must be applied two to three times a day. Sometimes, a two or three re-touch procedures are necessary.

CHAPTER 27

COSMETIC DENTISTRY:

To Complete the Picture with a Close-to-Perfect Smile

By Dudley Cheu, D.D.S.

I can remember growing up wishing that I and everyone I knew had a smile like Farrah Fawcett's. What an incredible smile!

A pretty smile is a nice addition to facial harmony and balance. A chipped tooth, tooth discoloration, or missing teeth can catch your eye. Today, with the development of several new techniques in cosmetic dentistry, amazing techniques can fix these imperfections and create beautiful smiles.

Plastic surgeons also treat patients who have been in bad car accidents where multiple teeth have been lost, and cosmetic dentistry becomes extremely important in restoring a person's smile.

A NEW GENERATION OF DENTISTRY

For the person who wishes to change his smile, cosmetic dentistry today offers many natural-looking alternatives to the silver amalgam fillings and the porcelain-fused-to-metal crowns.

With the new generation of all porcelain crowns, the problems of black lines at the gum line of old crowns are eliminated along with any tissue sensitivity to

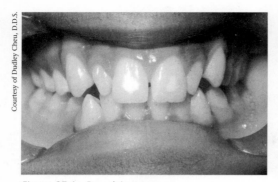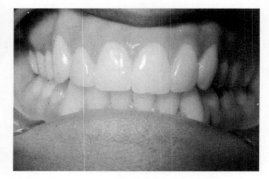

Courtesy of Dudley Cheu, D.D.S.

Figure 27-1. Porcelain veneers

metals. These crowns have a natural teeth-like appearance and function and perform like natural dentition. They have the same durability and wearability of natural enamel and the fit is extremely precise.

Porcelain and Composite Resins

Porcelain and composite resins offer aesthetic alternatives to unsightly silver amalgam fillings. These new restorations wear like natural teeth and will not damage opposing tooth structure. Needing only minimal tooth preparation, they are apt to preserve a more healthy tooth. The fillings have ideal anatomical contour and fit so they will look and feel like your natural teeth. Best of all, because they are bonded to the teeth, they will restore the tooth to nearly its original strength. All concerns of mercury leakage and unsightly metal appearance are eliminated, as the patient receives a highly natural aesthetic restoration with very good durability. It would be hard to determine your real tooth from one of the new restorations.

The "Perfect" Smile . . . Cheshire Cat Mode

For the anterior teeth, which are most visible in smiling, porcelain veneers are the restoration of choice. Veneers may solve common problems, including gaps between teeth, discolored or faulty fillings, eroded teeth, fractured and chipped teeth, and malaligned uneven teeth. The veneers look and feel natural and have exceptional fit to the teeth. Minimal tooth preparation is necessary, and the veneer will also strengthen the tooth because it is bonded with a tight seal to the facial aspect of the tooth. In two appointments, you can have whiter teeth with ideal size and shape to fit your new smile. Porcelain veneers offer optimal aesthetics because they are highly polished with an incredible smooth surface and are extremely color stable.

Bleaching

For minor aesthetic concerns, the dentist can cosmetically contour teeth to decrease the appearance of overcrowding or unevenness. Periodontists can reposition, graft, and recontour receding gums to restore them back to healthy-looking tissues. Finally, custom bleaching can whiten teeth that need no other dental restorations.

Dental Implants for Missing Teeth

In more complicated and involved cases, dental implants can replace missing teeth. Orthodontics can align severely crowded and malaligned dentitions. Oral and maxillofacial surgery can reposition the upper or lower jaw, and finally, plastic surgery can greatly enhance the shape of a smile by addressing wrinkling and sagging facial tissue around the lips.

Dudley Cheu, D.D.S., is a practicing dentist in San Francisco.

CHAPTER 28

Skin Care Products:

Retin-A and Alphahydroxy Acids

M ost likely, you've heard of Retin-A and alphahydroxy acids (AHAs) lately, and that they've been found to be beneficial to skin care, but how many of you really know what these AHAs are and how you use them?

The use of AHAs to "manage" age is a rediscovery of an age-old remedy. (It actually dates back to Cleopatra's time.) The most talked-about ingredients on the skin-care scene today are derived from nature—grapes, apples, lemons, passion fruit. Sound like a dieter's delight? In fact, these staples, along with sugar cane, sour milk, and aged wine are a natural source of citrus, glycolic, lactic, and tartaric acids. Falling into the category of alphahydroxy acids, these natural substances were researched by the scientific community about fifteen years ago. What scientists discovered was that AHAs act as natural exfoliators, sloughing away dead cells that build up on the topmost layer of skin. In doing so, surface lines, age spots, and uneven pigmentation are lightened. Unlike Retin-A, use of the AHAs will not result in excessive reddening, flaking, and sun sensitivity, and most everyone can benefit from using these products.

In actuality, many of my patients inquire about face-lifts when, in fact, their skin is really the problem. A face-lift can tighten skin that's sagging, but it will not correct the look of the skin itself. This is why I perform chemical skin peels using alphahydroxy acids either in conjunction with face-lifts or by themselves. However, if a patient wants to do an at-home chemical peel, I highly recommend combining a 10 percent solution of alphahydroxy acid with a specially formulated facial moisturizer. The program is very effective as a superficial peeling agent to smooth the skin and alleviate such conditions as fine wrinkles, sun-damaged skin (the weathered look), dry skin, acne, and blotchy pigmentation.

The lactic acid allows the exfoliation, or shedding, of outer dry skin layers which then causes and increases the turnover rate of new, younger dermal layer cells. Most patients report that with continual use of the system, they experience an improvement in broken capillaries, large pores, and acne. Since this system uses lactic acid, which is predominate in animal systems, it will, therefore, account for better results on human skin. As a plastic surgeon who understands the structure and function of both healthy and damaged skin, I am confident about the results.

There are many advantages in using alphahydroxy acids. It is less harsh on the skin than Retin-A, and separating the fruit acid cleanser from the moisturizer allows those with excessive dryness to use more moisturizer. The products rarely cause sensitivity to sunlight, and there is no need for missed work due to healing time.

If you want to improve the appearance of your skin by greatly reducing fine wrinkles, spots, pigmentation changes, acne, blotches, and by restoring the soft, natural feel of youthful skin, I highly recommend products containing alphahydroxy.

CHAPTER 29

WHAT CAN GO WRONG:

The Complications of Plastic Surgery

Complications from plastic surgery occur very rarely; however, if they do, they can be remedied, so do not despair. You have teamed up with your surgeon for the full duration. Prior to undergoing operation, your surgeon should thoroughly outline all of the possible risks and complications that may occur with your particular procedure. Understand them well, and ask your surgeon what he or she would need to do if something should happen.

Remember, you are in agreement together, and you, too, must assume some responsibility for your surgery. This means following all directions, going to your postoperative appointments, not smoking, avoiding heavy lifting, sleeping with your head elevated, massaging your scar religiously with vitamin E when necessary, and taking the full course of antibiotics. Most importantly, call your doctor when something doesn't seem right. If a complication occurs, your surgeon will sit down with you and discuss a game plan, whether it is a course of antibiotics, a touch-up procedure, or a return to the operating room to control bleeding.

The majority of complications are treatable, resulting in good to excellent outcomes, so keep this in mind. In this section I will outline the specific complications that can occur for each plastic surgery procedure. Most complications, however, can be narrowed down to three: bleeding, infection, and scarring.

BLEEDING

This complication can occur for a few reasons. It is very important to discontinue any aspirin-containing products at least two weeks prior to any procedure (see the list on page 41). Taking something as simple as Alka-Seltzer right before your elective operation can be a big problem. If you have high blood pressure you may be a setup for postoperative bleeding. Make sure you are continuing to take your medication even after your surgery, unless your physician recommends that you specifically do not need it. Increased activity can also be a big culprit. I remember one man who went waterskiing right after a nose surgery. He developed major bleeding from his nose requiring admission to the hospital for three days and a blood transfusion. Your surgeon will obtain a bleeding time and other related blood tests prior to your procedure to check your coagulation ability.

If bleeding occurs, your worst-case scenario is an immediate return to the operating room to control bleeding, evacuate any clot, and re-close the incisions. Generally speaking, your final result should not be affected.

So, to limit your chance of bleeding from the operative site make sure you discontinue all aspirin-containing products, take your blood pressure medications if you are on them, and limit your activity postoperatively.

INFECTIONS

Infection generally presents itself as redness with an associated fever. Watch for this, and report any change to your doctor immediately. Infections may occur up to 5 percent of the time with all operations. Most plastic surgeons realize this and recommend antibiotics before the operation as well as after to prevent this. I think that plastic surgeons are superstitious when it comes to infections. Perhaps, at times, antibiotics are over-prescribed. If you should develop an infection that is not responsive to oral antibiotics your doctor may prescribe intravenous antibiotics which can now be administered at home rather than in a hospital setting.

SCARRING

Scarring is a concern with all operations. Your own personal history of how your skin responded to a specific injury will predict how you respond to an elective cosmetic operation. Incisions will go through a series of transitions as they are healing. Initially after about two weeks they may look pretty good; at about six weeks, due to the collagen buildup around the scar, the healing incision will look red, raised, lumpy, and bumpy. Don't be discouraged. This is the normal healing process. Most plastic surgeons are very meticulous in their closures of incisions; they know what makes a good scar and what doesn't. Trust them, and trust the healing process. By about three to six months, the incisions will begin their maturation process. A scar will look much better at one year and even better at two years. Try to be patient during the process.

The location of the incision is also a predictor of what it will look like. Scars on the back, shoulders, elbows, and knees will heal with generally wider scars than incisions of the upper eyelids. Your surgeon will be the barometer during the healing process. Steroid injections in the scar, vitamin E oil, Silastic sheeting, or even laser can help improve the look of scars.

COMPLICATIONS FOLLOWING RHYTIDECTOMY, OR FACE-LIFT

In addition to the three most common complications following face-lifts, there may be sensory nerve injury, motor nerve injury, skin necrosis, postoperative swelling, skin changes, hair loss contour deformities, earlobe differences, change in your hairline, early recurrence of deformity, and patient dissatisfaction.

Now let's review each of these individually. If a hematoma does develop (swelling under the skin of the face related to bleeding), your surgeon will need to either aspirate the area with a needle and syringe if it is small, or, he will need to take you back into the operating room and remove the hematoma and reclose your incision. Your final result will not be affected.

If you opt for a deep plane face-lift, such as a SMAS (superficial musculo aponeurotic system) rhytidectomy or a subperiosteal face-lift, you are at possible risk for loss of facial muscle function due to loss of a motor nerve branch. There is quite a bit of "crossover" with regard to the nerve supply to the face. If one small branch is cut during the face-lift in the cheek region, there will be several other neighborhood nerves that will take over the territory and provide function. Sometimes right after an operation the patient will have a weak smile on one side of the face. This is common, and expect it to improve within three to four months. Sometimes it may take up to a year to improve. There are two other nerves that plastic surgeons need to watch out for: the frontalis branch and the marginal mandibular branch. The first allows you to raise your eyebrow, and the latter provides function to your lower lip. If either of these are injured during a face-lift, return of function is possible, but rare.

Skin necrosis can occur in people who smoke around the time of their operation. Nicotine from cigarettes constrict the tiny blood vessels causing a decrease in the blood supply to the area. Even the popular nicotine patches can cause problems with wound healing after a face-lift. The most common location for necrosis is the area right behind the ear and, occasionally, in front of the ear. If you don't smoke, then don't worry about this problem. If you do smoke, quit at least a couple of weeks before you have face-lift surgery. The area behind the ear will turn black and form a hard scab the size of a dime or a silver dollar.

Eventually the area will heal, but it will take a while, maybe three to four weeks of time. During this period your plastic surgeon will have you do daily dressing changes in the area.

Swelling

Swelling is normal in all patients after face-lift procedures. The majority of surgeons recommend that their patients keep their face elevated during the healing process. I usually have my patients sleep on four to six pillows for the first week, and reduce it to two to four the following week. I do not recommend ice on the skin of the face unless I have done an eyelid procedure. If so, I allow ice only on the eyelid area and in no other place.

Infection

Because the blood supply to the face is so good, the possibility of an infection following a face-lift is very uncommon. However, in all of my patients I cover them with antibiotics before, during, and after any face-lift procedure. The most common infection, if it does occur, is a staph or strep infection. Common signs and symptoms will include redness, swelling, tenderness, and heat over the skin involved. Once treated the infection resolves, and there is generally little to no effect on your final result.

Skin Changes

Patients with darker skin, high risk of bruising, and overexposure to ultraviolet light are set up to develop hyperpigmentation, or dark pigmentation of the skin, in the area of the face-lift. The condition may require the use of chemical peels or makeup following the procedure. This condition is rare.

Scarring

The incision for a face-lift begins in front of the ear, and travels behind the ear. The incision in front of the ear heals very well. The incision behind the ear can result in a scar which, according to most patients, does not heal as well. However, most patient's hairstyles are such that they hide these incisions very well.

If a scar is raised, red, and noticeable it can be improved upon by using steroid injections, laser, or Silastic sheeting. "Tincture of Time," or waiting it out, also improves the look of these scars.

Hair Loss

If the incision for the face-lift extends up into the temple area of the scalp, and/or in the hairline behind the ear, a patient is at risk for transient injury to the hair follicles. The loss is usually noticed about two to three weeks postoperatively. Regrowth of the hair follicles takes place within fourteen weeks. Patients who smoke or have thin hair are at risk for this problem.

Ear Lobe Deformity

Every plastic surgeon who is properly trained in the procedure of rhytidectomy will aim to prevent what we call in the profession a "pixie ear." This is where the earlobe is sewn to a point lower on the face than where it was intended to be. It is relatively easy to correct and can be done by your surgeon under local anesthesia.

Discomfort

Pain after this procedure is very uncommon. Many sensory fibers are essentially asleep after the operation. Many of my patients don't even take pain medication afterward. It is common to have nonspecific shooting pains and itching afterward. Immediately after the procedure, my patients may complain of feeling sort of "tight." This is common, and it improves considerably during the first week.

Patient Dissatisfaction

Patients who express dissatisfaction after face-lift surgery do so mainly because they had unrealistic expectations of what plastic surgery can really do. It wasn't what they expected. Expectations are really key here. Many patients who have undergone previous plastic surgery understand and know the process. They understand the initial swelling period, the bruising period, and the healing process of the incisions. They know what to say to their friends and relatives and what their reactions are going to be. The more supportive your network of friends, relatives, husbands, and wives, the better.

COMPLICATIONS FOLLOWING BLEPHAROPLASTY

Before a surgeon performs eyelid surgery or blepharoplasty surgery, she will ask you several questions about your health, your ophthalmologic history (how have your eyes been), and whether your eyes are usually dry. You may be asked to see an ophthalmologist ahead of time to have a thorough evaluation before proceeding with any type of surgery.

The complications that can occur following this type of procedure are bleeding, infection, and scarring. Additionally, you may end up with dry eyes requiring frequent eye drops for a few months.

There may be inadequate resection of fatty tissue that requires repeat touch-up revision—excess skin which was not excised with the initial operation or retraction of the lids due to excessive excision of skin tissue, later requiring a skin graft. Occasionally, though very rarely, there may be injury to the cornea due to exposure; keratitis; or a problem with the drainage due to swelling. Although extremely rare, visual loss can occur but is very uncommon.

Bleeding, infection, and scarring are all treatable. A repeat operation can take care of excess fat or skin. If for any reason after your blepharoplasty you develop tightness around your eyelids and difficulty with your vision, your plastic surgeon needs to know immediately.

COMPLICATIONS FOLLOWING RHINOPLASTY

Most complications related to rhinoplasty can be included in the "main 3"—bleeding, infection, scarring—and poor healing. In general, finding out what your nose will look like after surgery will take several weeks to several months. Be patient. A small bump of scar tissue may show up at three months. It may resolve, or it may become more prominent requiring a touch-up procedure down the road.

Plastic surgeons tend to do minor touch-up operations to improve a nose following a rhinoplasty at least 17 to 25 percent of the time.

Sometimes a patient will feel small lumps and bumps on the surface of the skin that are not visible but easily felt. Probably every single patient of a rhinoplasty will have a few irregularities. If they are not visible, be patient. They may resolve. If they are visible, your doctor can do a touch-up procedure once all healing has taken place.

Breast Surgery

Breast Augmentation
The risks and complications were carefully reviewed in the section on breast augmentation. See Chapter 12.

Breast Reduction/Mastopexy
Probably of most concern to patients following this operation are the incisions. However, most women undergoing breast reductions care little about the scars. They are glad their breasts are smaller—their back pain has improved, and they feel better.

Occasionally, especially if a woman smokes cigarettes, there can be problems with the blood supply to the nipples. This is very rare. If there is complete loss of blood supply to the nipples, a nipple reconstruction will need to be performed.

Abdominoplasty

The incision after abdominoplasty can take months to look reasonable—usually about twelve months. Again, most patients are so happy with the improvement that they are not bothered by the redness of the incision. Your surgeon will show you pictures of incisions, and perhaps let you talk to a few patients to prepare you for your recovery.

Before surgery, many patients will joke with me about the position of their belly button making sure that I'll put it in the right place. The majority of plastic surgeons that perform this operation are highly trained and familiar with abdominoplasty. Those that are well-trained consider this operation to be rather straightforward, so making sure that the belly button is in the right location is relatively easy. There have been a few lawsuits settled for placing the belly button in the wrong location, but this has usually occurred in cases performed by non-certified surgeons.

LIPOSUCTION

Liposuction is a relatively easy operation that usually goes smoothly with minimal problems. However, bleeding and infection may occur. Bruising under the skin is a normal part of the healing process and will take three to four weeks to dissipate.

If there is significant bleeding or an unusual amount of swelling, notify your surgeon immediately as this may indicate a hematoma. Your surgeon may be able to aspirate to remove some of this fluid.

The small incisions will remain permanent scars. Waviness of the skin can also occur, especially if cellulite is present. It is very difficult to eliminate cellulite with liposuction, so don't expect this to go away. Swelling can persist for up to six months, and it may take this long to see the final results.

Shock requiring blood transfusion is rare, especially with the new temescent technique. Transfusions were once necessary when more than 1,500 ccs of fat were removed.

A fat embolus is an extremely rare complication. Symptoms for this include shortness of breath and a general sense of illness. Contact doctor your immediately if you develop these symptoms.

Repeat touch-up procedures are common after liposuction, and you may want to consider one.

HOW WILL MY SURGEON HANDLE MY COMPLICATION IF IT DOES OCCUR?

Most surgeons are just as concerned as you are about a complication, maybe even more so. They want everything to go as smoothly and as perfectly as you do, but complications do happen. If something doesn't seem right . . . you don't feel well, you have a lot of swelling on one side of your face-lift, your left breast implant seems quite a lot larger than the right, you've spiked a temperature to 102 degrees, contact your doctor *immediately*. Every single one of these worst-case scenarios has a cure.

If there is a hematoma or evidence of bleeding following a face-lift, breast augmentation, or any of the other procedures, it will require at most a one-hour procedure to open the incision, control the bleeding, and re-close the incision. Your final result will not be affected. If there is infection, your doctor will put you on antibiotics until the infection clears.

Scarring is unpredictable. We have been doing the majority of these operations for the last ten to thirty years using pretty much the same types of incisions (some we've been doing since 3000 B.C.). Scar management is one of the most highly researched areas in our field. Plastic surgery continues to make significant advances in this area, especially now with laser surgery.

Although complications with any operation are possible, remember, they're uncommon. Otherwise, plastic surgery wouldn't be popular. The majority of patients are very happy with their result. Realistic expectations play a key role in postoperative recovery. Remember, your plastic surgeon is seeking "perfection" always, but realistically, plastic surgery is improvement, not perfection.

REVISIONARY OR TOUCH-UP PROCEDURES

At times you or your plastic surgeon will notice something after an operation, something that just didn't heal the way you hoped: the nipple shifted some and needs to be remedied; your nose developed some scar tissue and the scar tissue needs to be removed; one breast implant seems a little bigger than the other; and a million other reasons.

At this point both you and your surgeon need to decide if it's worth doing a "touch-up" procedure. Some patients can be quite extreme, hoping for perfection, and requesting it every step of the way. If the patient's request for improvement is realistic, and I feel that I can make it better, I will recommend a small revision. If not, I sit down with them and discuss realistic expectations as I do before all procedures. I will often refer them to other plastic surgeons for a second and third opinion. Sometimes hearing input from two or three physicians, can help a patient feel more comfortable with the final result.

In our community, we have a plastic surgery society which meets once a month to discuss plastic surgery cases. It's a wonderful service to the patient as well as to the plastic surgeon. The patient gets the benefit of multiple opinions in one visit and new ideas, perhaps not considered by the primary surgeon, are discussed and considered.

At any rate, it is not unusual for your surgeon to recommend a "touch-up" procedure especially if something is bothering you about the outcome, or if he feels that they can make it better.

The surgeon will usually do these minor touch-up procedures at no charge, but you will be required to pay for the supplies, anesthesia, if necessary, and the operating room, if used.

CHAPTER 30

OTHER TIMES I MAY NEED THE SERVICES OF A PLASTIC SURGEON:

Trauma, Breast Reconstruction, Hand Surgery, Congenital Birth Defects

When people think of plastic surgery they often think of face-lifts and movie stars. They are often surprised when we show up at an emergency room on a Saturday night to help repair facial lacerations sustained during a fall or a car accident. Michael Jackson met his plastic surgeon after he was burned while filming a commercial for Coca-Cola.

We are fully trained surgeons who have had many years of general surgery training as well as plastic surgery training. I have learned to think of a plastic surgeon as the Renaissance surgeon, as we are trained in many aspects of surgery. The reason why plastic surgery is so appealing to many surgeons is that it is very diverse and creative and challenging. Many plastic surgeons after their training will specialize in a certain aspect within the field such as hand surgery or microsurgery or specifically cosmetic surgery. Some surgeons will specialize in just noses. Others specialize in only breast surgery, such as breast reconstruction following mastectomy.

A couple of years ago a young man was involved in an awful accident with a large piece of farming equipment. He sustained complete amputation of both his arms below the elbow. A team of plastic surgeons and orthopedic surgeons were involved with the reattachment of his limbs. He is currently doing quite well and is grateful for their help.

Several times a year plastic surgeons donate their time and surgical skills to countries abroad who have limited resources and few plastic surgeons to help take care of individuals with cleft lips and cleft palates, burn injuries, war injuries, or complex medical problems. During my training, one of my professors took care of an orphan girl with severe scar contractures from a burn injury. She was unable to move her arm which had become attached to her chest wall due to a severe burn scar. A special operation which repositioned the muscle from her back allowed the surgeon to free her arm, and she was able to use it once again. She was eventually brought to this country and was adopted by a very close friend of the plastic surgeon.

Some of the organizations involved with helping abroad are Rotoplast and Operation Smile, among others. If you would be interested in helping on any of these trips and you have a medical background you may contact the organization, and they will direct you to someone in charge.

During my training I was exposed to an extensive array of complex operative procedures for young children born with severe craniofacial abnormalities—children with cleft lips and palates and some with orbits set very far apart (called hypertelorism), children with multiple digits, some born without a thumb, some without a nose. There were many children who were taken care of by the cranio-facial service at Rush Presbyterian in Chicago where I trained. It was a very rewarding time for me, a time I will never forget.

You can see whether you meet "one of us" in our office in consultation for a face-lift or in the emergency room to repair your six-year-old's laceration from a bicycle accident. . . . It is all in the name of plastic surgery.

The Age Wave:

Improvement Not Perfection

"So, did you have a good vacation? You look so rested."

This is a perfect comment for the recovering plastic surgery patient to hear. Your goal was to look better, more rested, refreshed, and, of course, younger. But you didn't want the whole world to know just how you accomplished your fabulous new look. Good plastic surgery makes you look better, not "done." If someone says, "Oh, what a wonderful face-lift!" then it wasn't. If your new eyes make you look like you are always frightened, then the surgeon overdid it. These are a few more reasons for a good discussion with your doctor at the consultation, demonstrating that you have come prepared and that you are aware that these things can happen. Once the surgery is done, however, there isn't much, short of additional surgery, that can be done to correct the problems. Makeup and hairstyles can help, and, with time, the skin's elasticity is naturally reduced so that the desired results will come eventually.

Actually, most patients are ecstatic about their new face, nose, body, breasts, etc., and can experience a wide range of emotions. There are those patients who are so elated that they can hardly contain themselves, while others are a little more subdued and are not quite ready to be scrutinized by the public. In the past, plastic surgery was kept a secret, a luxury that one never admitted, but still indulged in to thwart the ravages of time. Then, along came Phyllis Diller who has had most pro-cedures known to man (and admits it), and all of a sudden plastic surgery was out of the closet! It is now considered a very acceptable way to soften the blow of time, and, as we mentioned in Chapter 3, thousands of procedures are performed each year.

So, you are one of many! You've finally had the surgery that you've always wanted, and, all of a sudden, the world looks different. Some patients find them-selves walking with a little more energy in their step, while some gaze at their reflection in the mirror longer than usual.

Remember that important presentation that you're scheduled to make to your firms biggest client? Perhaps your confidence has just taken a major leap, and you'll feel so much more self-assured when you step into that meeting room. We are not suggesting that your new look will win you accounts at the office, but often the patients who have had the surgery they wanted suddenly feel more secure with themselves and with their abilities. Some executives feel that looking more youth-ful has advantages when dealing with other professionals. In our youth-conscious society some business people feel that there are disadvantages to looking older, and many opt for plastic surgery.

Many women who have worked at home raising children and organized a multitude of lives and events for most of their years find that plastic surgery gives them a whole new outlook on things. All of a sudden, maybe mid-life isn't so bad! After all those years of cooking, bathing little ones, packing lunches, carpooling, PTA meetings, and watching endless plays, concerts, and sporting events, the "new" person looking back in the mirror looks pretty darn good.

Even teenagers, who have not experienced the ravages of time or an accumu-lation of life's experiences, can find that reshaping a nose or reducing the size of large breasts can immediately make life more pleasant. Older patients can benefit enormously and often feel invigorated, more youthful, and have added emotional energy after their surgeon has erased ten to fifteen years off their appearance.

No matter who the patient is, the majority of plastic surgery patients who have chosen to change some physical characteristics with themselves are pleased with the results. They've been improved, but not perfected, and they knew that this was their goal all along. After all, "perfect" has no character, no individuality, no distinction. Your surgery has simply improved you and made you better than you were (at least on the outside). Isn't that what you wanted from the start?

We have come to the end of our book, and we truly hope that you are now thoroughly prepared if you are considering plastic surgery. We have tried to anticipate your concerns and questions and, hopefully, have addressed them all. If you have further questions, we suggest calling your local medical society, the American Medical Society, or the American Society of Plastic and Reconstructive Surgeons. We sincerely wish you good health and great pleasure and contentment with your plastic surgery experience.

SHOULD I *REALLY* DO THIS?

By Carolyn J. Cline, M.D., Ph.D.

I f you are contemplating plastic surgery, one of the questions you undoubtedly have on your mind is, "Should I *really* do this?" During more than a decade of private practice as a plastic surgeon I have found that people can go around and around with this question for days, weeks, months, and even years because the question itself contains many hidden agendas. The major clue to what is going on with this question is the word "should." What does it really mean? Does it mean, "Is it safe?" or, "Can I afford it?"

The question that troubles people is, "Is it personally, morally, and socially okay for me to do this?" Guilt often lurks beneath uncertainty. One of my patients confessed, "If I were the person I really should be, I wouldn't have to do this." Another, a graduate student, told me, "My friends will kill me if they find out. They think we should live with what God gave us." (I reminded her that God gave us cosmetic plastic surgeons, too!) Sixty-five-year-old Ann said, "I have the money, but I shouldn't spend it on something so frivolous as a face-lift. I could give the money to my grandson to buy a sportscar." (Talk about frivolous!) One gray-haired professor confided, "My mother would roll over in her grave if she knew I was here. I can still hear her voice: 'You're beautiful just the way you are. Stop looking in the mirror all the time; someday a man is going to appreciate you for who you really are.'"

Feelings of guilt have to be resolved before surgery for practical reasons. The unconscious can cause real trouble afterward. "Okay," it says, "you did it. But you shouldn't have, so I'm going to punish you." What kind of punishment? Jessica, a fifty-four-year-old lawyer experienced unexplained pain after her face-lift. The pain only resolved itself after she acknowledged her ambivalent feelings about not growing old gracefully. Another patient, Pamela, a twenty-five-year-old secretary, could not accept her breast implants as a part of herself after having a long-desired breast augmentation. She, too, was only able to accept them after she acknowledged her guilt over competitive feelings with her mother, who had larger breasts. Then there was Margaret, a thirty-eight-year-old nurse, who had diffuse guilt—guilt about being alive. The daughter of a holocaust victim, her basic philosophy toward life was, "It's okay if you do it, just as long as you do not enjoy it." A postoperative depression following her blepharoplasty and breast augmentation sent her into therapy. Later, she wrote me a letter in which she said that having her surgery was the best thing she'd ever done; not only did she love the way she looked, but she had been forced to confront lifelong issues and could finally be happy in life.

INNER TYRANTS

These are the voices that hold us back from doing what we want to do, even when we've been intelligent about gathering the pertinent information. These disguised voices of guilt work in devious ways. One forty-four-year-old woman became absolutely panic stricken just before her breast reduction surgery. Her anxiety was palpable. She was sure she was going to die, so we canceled the surgery. Later, it became clear that she felt she was going against her mother's advice and would therefore be punished. The fact that her mother was long deceased didn't matter. Her mother had always frowned upon doing things for the sake of vanity, and she was still struggling with letting her mother down.

Sometimes a group ethos becomes a tyrant. The women's movement, a phenomenon in which I participated and highly regard, has spawned a cadre of women who intensely disapprove of plastic surgery. From their point of view, a woman who undergoes such treatment falls prey to the wishes of a patriarchal society, interiorizing the male gaze. This constricting outlook decreases women's choices and, in fact, becomes a form of tyranny in itself. Berkeleyites by the drove have come into my office secretly, fearing lest their feminist friends get wind of it. I find this sad. Feminism is about increasing, not decreasing, women's options.

Another tyrannical group ethos uses the word vanity in conjunction with plastic surgery. That's another troublesome and ambiguous word. It is invoked in a pejorative way by those who disapprove of cosmetic surgery. Caring about your clothes, hair, makeup, and exercise is also a form of vanity, but somehow these things are okay. When it comes to surgery, though, vanity is the final bludgeon of the judgmental.

Vanity was believed by the Greeks to be a sister of Beauty and Justice and a virtue. What happened? Beauty was knocked from her pedestal by the sword of a well-intentioned but now outworn puritanical notion that attention paid to the body took something away from the soul. These principles are not mutually exclusive.

The idea of symptom replacement is another old saw. As a former psychologist, I remember a strong belief within the profession that wanting to change how one looked through surgery was seen as a symptom of an unresolved psychological issue, and once the change was achieved, something else would replace it as a cause of dissatisfaction. Unfortunately, this misconception survives today.

There is no real difference between cosmetic plastic surgery and reconstructive plastic surgery. We tend to think of the latter as acceptable because it is necessary. Discomfort with a body part that one is born with, or with an aging face which no longer reflects a youthful spirit, is just as deforming to the person who bears it as a scar from an accident.

BEAUTY

Whether we like it or not, appearance impacts us greatly. Our fast-paced society allows little time to get to know one another, so a first impression becomes a very powerful factor in making decisions about, say, courting or hiring. Psychological studies show that more attractive people are thought to be nicer, smarter, more competent, and more reliable. Unfortunately unfair, but true.

Over the fifteen years I've been in practice, the number of men undergoing plastic surgery has drastically increased. I see several interesting aspects to this phenomenon: Men are divorced more often and increasingly aware of the tentative nature of the job market even at the highest levels. Men trained to make executive decisions quickly learn to consider their own physiques as they would corporate bodies. Thus, it is useful to clarify, streamline, and market them, if you will. Men are simply putting their best foot forward, and their mothers would surely approve of that.

Beauty is a practical issue in our society. When people are uncomfortable with a body part, they feel deformed. And if they feel deformed, they act deformed. They are less assertive, less adventuresome, and sometimes reclusive. Often they settle for less in life, or do strange gymnastics to make a life. Before her rhinoplasty, Barbara would only approach people from a certain angle, lest they see her full profile. Eventually, growing obsessed, she limited not only others' point-of-view, but her own view of things through this angle. After her surgery, she exclaimed, "I had no idea how much time and energy I had bound up with trying to live with the nose I thought ugly. I feel so freed up now and so much more energetic."

MAKING THE DECISION

Most people seeking cosmetic surgery are very well adjusted. You are probably one of them. But if you have some guilty feelings lurking in the shadows, you can work with yourself to straighten them out. You can begin by becoming the critical voice that is telling you not to do it. Talk out loud. Say all the unspeakable things this voice has been whispering in your ear. Relish the experience. After all, this voice is *you*. Be forceful, even say the ridiculous if it comes into your mind. When you start to hear the voice that wants the surgery, switch to that voice. Give vent to your yearnings and wishes that voice is expressing. You may find that there is a third voice coming forth, a moderating voice, a dealmaker. That is your adult self who wants to negotiate between the other two voices. Speak the thoughts and feelings of the dealmaker. Repeat this process a few times. After a while, you will most likely be able to make peace amongst the warring parties. You may come to realize that the critical voice has been stopping you from doing a number of things in life. Good. You're on your way to positive change. If you can't make peace with yourself, counseling might help. On the whole, I have found that people are very creative dealmakers.

You will approach plastic surgery the way you approach most other new situations in your life. One common question people have is, "Should I do everything at once or one at a time?" Once the medical safety of any approach is established, the answer depends on your personality and style. Some people like to dive into the water; others like to put a toe in first, and enter gradually. Which type are you? This will give you a clue as to how you will most comfortably undergo surgery.

A fear that many have is that once they have plastic surgery, they'll never stop, sort of like eating nuts or potato chips. This fear, like most, is unfounded. Only once have I encountered a patient with a continual need to change his appearance. And I would not even consider him an addict, but someone who could not accept himself on a basic level. The vast majority of patients successfully undergo surgery and move on in life with more self-esteem, energy, and determination. As the husband of one of my patients said, "Before her surgery, Jeannie was wishy-washy about making decisions; now she just moves ahead. She even tells me off now and then which she never would do before. I kinda like it," he grinned.

There is such a phenomenon as total body discontent, and that can be solved only through psychological work. Joan, a thirty-seven-year-old decorator was a prime example. She came into my office saying "I hate my hips, I hate my thighs, I hate my breasts, I hate my face, I hate all of it." Joan was a poor candidate for plastic surgery. She was disgusted with being overweight and with her unsatisfying life over which she felt little control. She underwent counseling, lost sixty pounds, and emerged with a much more positive self-image. Only then could we surgically address her lack of upper and lower body proportion.

AM I A GOOD CANDIDATE?

You may be wondering: "How do I know if I am a good candidate for cosmetic plastic surgery?" If you like yourself generally but are bothered by a certain circumscribed area of the body, then it's worth seeking a cosmetic surgery consultation. Once you find that improvement is safe and possible, consider the following questions:

1. *What role do I expect plastic surgery to play in my life?*
   Be sure your expectations are reasonable. Cosmetic surgical change will not bring you a boyfriend if your personality is unpleasant; it won't bring you

a job if you are unskilled or unkempt; and it won't keep a wandering husband close to home.

2. *Have I truly resolved my ambivalent feelings?*
For instance, do you still hear an invisible voice ringing in your ears, "You're so vain, and all this money you're spending, it's a sin." Resolve the conflict by talking with yourself out loud so that you can be one hundred percent behind what you're doing.

3. *Have I dealt with the significant others in my life who disapprove of cosmetic surgery?*
Settle the issue with them, perhaps through the gentle assertion that it's none of their business. You've already settled it for yourself. The last thing you'll want to hear when you're recovering is undermining, guilt-provoking comments from others. During your postoperative period. you need tender loving care not criticism.

4. *How will I cope with a complication if I get one?*
Chances are you won't get one. But if you are one of the rare birds who does, you need to be able to say to yourself and mean it: "I will not criticize myself for undergoing this surgery. I went about this procedure thoughtfully and intelligently. That's all I could ask of myself. I'm glad I did it because I really wanted to, and I'll live through this period and be kind and gentle with myself."

Choosing a good doctor is key to a successful outcome. You need someone who is not only qualified but who really listens to you and cares about you. The first step in finding a good plastic surgeon is to find someone who is board certified or board eligible in the specialty. The American Society of Plastic and Reconstructive Surgeons will give you the names of three qualified surgeons in your area. Interview them. Ask to talk to former patients. See if you feel listened to; trust your reactions. If it doesn't feel right, this person isn't right for you. Move on and find someone who not only does good work but is someone with whom you feel rapport. You will be living with the results of your surgery, not the doctor. Look carefully after your own well-being. If you do, chances are you will have an extremely rewarding experience.

Carolyn J. Cline, M.D., Ph.D., is a board-certified plastic and reconstructive surgeon practicing for more than a decade in San Francisco. Prior to her establishing her surgical practice, she was a successful psychotherapist. Dr. Cline is a graduate of Wellesley College, Harvard University, and Washington University, and she completed her surgical training at Stanford and St. Francis Hospitals in San Francisco. A leading authority on the effect of cosmetic change on psychological well-being, Dr. Cline frequently appears as a guest expert on national television.

RESOURCES

American Society of Plastic and
  Reconstructive Surgeons
444 E. Algonquin Road
Arlington Heights, IL 60005
Phone: (847) 228-9000
1-800-635-0635

American Board of Plastic Surgeons, Inc.
Steve Penn Center, Suite 400
35 Market Street
Philadelphia, PA 19103
Phone: (215) 587-9322

American Society for Aesthetic Plastic
  Surgeons, Inc.
444 E. Algonquin Road
Arlington Heights, IL 60005
Phone: (847) 228-9274

The American Medical Association
515 North State Street
Chicago, IL 60610
Phone: (312) 464-5000

The American Academy of Facial Plastic
  and Reconstructive Surgery
1101 Vermont Avenue, N.W.
Suite 404, Dept. MC
Washington, D.C. 20005
Phone: 1-800-332-3223

Also contact your local medical society and
hospitals and medical centers in your area.

GLOSSARY OF TERMS

Abdominoplasty: A "tummy tuck" where muscles in the abdomen are tightened and excess skin is removed

Augmentation Mammoplasty: Insertion of an implant to enlarge the breast

Blepharoplasty: Eyelid surgery which removes fat, excess skin, and muscle from the upper and lower eyelids

Breast Reconstruction: Creating a new breast after mastectomy or trauma

Browplasty: The lifting of the brows and forehead to smooth skin, raise the upper eyelids, and minimize frown lines

Chemabrasion: A chemical peel using burning chemicals to uncover smoother skin

Dermabrasion: Use of a wire brush or other device to remove the outer layer of skin

Genioplasty: Contouring of the chin where fat is trimmed and underlying muscle is tightened

Laser resurfacing: Treatments using carbon dioxide (CO) to quickly vaporize cells on the skin's surface, erasing wrinkles, scars, and sun damage

Mastopexy: A breast lift, in which the nipple is repositioned and excess skin is removed

Mentoplasty: Chin augmentation with a solid implant, improving the profile by changing the size of the chin

Reduction Mammoplasty: Removal of skin and tissue to reduce the size of the breast

Rhinoplasty: The moving and shaping of bone, cartilage, and skin to change the appearance of the nose

Rhytidectomy: A face-lift, where the removal of excess fat, the tightening of underlying muscles, and the redraping of skin improve the signs of aging

BIBLIOGRAPHY

"Aesthetic Surgery of the Facial Skeleton," *Clinics in Plastic Surgery* vol. 18, no. 1. January 1971.

Alster, Tina, and David Apfelberg. *Cosmetic Laser Surgery*. New York: Wiley & Sons, 1996.

Baker, T. J., and H. L. Gordon. *Surgical Rejuvenation of the Face*. St. Louis: C.V. Mosby, 1985.

Barrett, B.M. Jr., ed. *Manual for Patient Care in Plastic Surgery*. Boston: Little, Brown, 1982.

"Blepharoplasty and Periorbital Aesthetic Surgery," *Clinics in Plastic Surgery* vol. 20, no. 2. April 1993.

Broadbent, T. R., and M. Woolf. "Rhinoplasty," in *Aesthetic Surgery,* edited by H. Courtiss. St. Louis: C.V. Mosby.

Curtis, E. H., ed. *Male Aesthetic Surgery*. St. Louis: C.V. Mosby, 1990.

"Dermatology for Plastic Surgery," *Clinics in Plastic Surgery* vol. 20, no. 11. January 1993.

Dudley, Hugh, and David Carter. *Rob & Smith's Operative Surgery*. 4th ed. London: Butterworth's, 1983.

Georgiade, N. G., ed. *Essentials of Plastic, Maxillofacial, and Reconstructive Surgery,* 2d ed. Baltimore: Williams & Wilkins, 1994.

————, G. S. Georgiade, and R. Riefkol. *Aesthetic Surgery of the Breast.* Philadelphia: W.B. Saunders, 1990.

Goin, J.M., and M.K. Goin. *Changing the Body: Psychological Effects of Plastic Surgery.* Baltimore: Williams & Wilkins, 1981.

Goldwyn, R.M. *The Patient and the Plastic Surgeon.* Boston: Little, Brown, 1981.

————, ed. *Reduction Mammoplasty.* Boston: Little, Brown, 1990.

————, ed. *The Unfavorable Result in Plastic Surgery, Avoidance and Treatment,* 2nd ed. Boston: Little, Brown, 1984.

Grabb, C., and J.W. Smith, eds. *Plastic Surgery,* 3rd ed. Boston: Little, Brown, 1979.

Grazer, F.M., and W.G. Wood. *Atlas of Body Contouring and Suction Assisted Lipectomy.* New York: Churchill Livingstone, 1992.

Habal, M., ed. *Advances in Plastic and Reconstructive Surgery,* vol. 6. Chicago: Year Book Medical, 1990.

Johnson, Calvin. *Open Structure Rhinoplasty.* Philadelphia: W.B. Saunders, 1990.

Jurkiewicz, M.J., et al. *Plastic Surgery Principles and Practice.* St. Louis: C.V. Mosby, 1990.

Kaye, B.L. *Facial Rejuvenative Surgery: A Color Photographic Atlas.* Philadelphia: J.B. Lippincott, 1987.

————, and G.P. Bradinger, eds. *Symposium on Problems and Complications in Aesthetic Plastic Surgery of the Face.* St. Louis: C.V. Mosby, 1984.

"Lipoplasty," *Clinics in Plastic Surgery* vol. 16, no. 2. April 1989.

"Male Aesthetic Surgery," *Clinics in Plastic Surgery* vol. 18, no. 4. October 1991.

McCarthy, John. *Plastic Surgery,* vols. 1–8. Philadelphia: W.B. Saunders, 1990.

McKinney, P., and B.L. Cunningham. *Aesthetic Facial Surgery.* New York: Churchill Livingston, 1992.

The Official Journal of the American Society of Plastic and Reconstructive Surgeons. Baltimore: Williams & Wilkins, 1985–1996.

Osler Institute Review Course. Philadelphia, 1993.

Papel, I.D., N.E. Nachlas, eds. *Facial and Reconstructive Surgery.* St. Louis: C.V. Mosby, 1992.

PDR, 1996.

Peck, George C., and G.C. Peck, Jr. *Complications and Problems in Aesthetic Plastic Surgery.* London: Gower Medical Publishing, 1992.

"Plastic and Reconstructive Surgery Journal," *The Official Journal of Plastic and Reconstructive Surgeons.* Baltimore: Williams & Wilkins, 1985-1996.

Rees, T.D., C. Baker, and N. Tabbal, eds. *Rhinoplasty: Problems and Controversies.* St. Louis: C.V. Mosby, 1988.

Regnault, P., and R. Daniel, eds. *Aesthetic Plastic Surgery.* Boston: Little Brown, 1984.

Sheen, J.H. *Aesthetic Rhinoplasty,* 2d ed. St. Louis: C.V. Mosby, 1987

Stanford Plastic Surgery Review Course. Stanford, Calif., 1994.

Terino, Ed. *Chin and Malar Augmentation.* London: Gower Medical Publishing, 1992.

Toddy, M.E., J.R. Thomas, and R.J. Brown. *Facial Aesthetic Surgery.* St. Louis: C.V. Mosby, 1995.

INDEX